Douglas H. Ruben, PhD

Writing for Money in Mental Health

Pre-publication
REVIEWS,
COMMENTARIES,
EVALUATIONS . . .

"**D**r. Ruben has done it again! He has written a timely, comprehensive, and informative book for mental health professionals in private practice who are struggling against the vicissitudes of the present mental health delivery system. This book is a must for any practitioner interested in earning extra income not regulated and controlled by the present requirements for mental health services.

This book provides timely and helpful hints to more efficiently market our services, change our self-image regarding our worth, and expand our imagination concerning new and various market ideas and techniques.

I strongly recommend this to any private practitioner who is attempting to survive and thrive in the rapidly and drastically changing mental health market."

Winfred J. Smith, PhD
Psychologist; Director,
Hope Counseling Center,
Lansing, MI

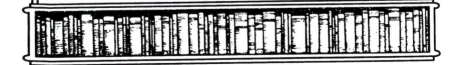

The Haworth Press, Inc.

Writing for Money in Mental Health

HAWORTH Marketing Resources
Innovations in Practice & Professional Services
William J. Winston, Senior Editor

New, Recent, and Forthcoming Titles:

Church and Ministry Strategic Planning: From Concept to Success by R. Henry Migliore, Robert E. Stevens, and David L. Loudon

Business in Mexico: Managerial Behavior, Protocol, and Etiquette by Candace Bancroft McKinniss and Arthur A. Natella

Managed Service Restructuring in Health Care: A Strategic Approach in a Competitive Environment by Robert L. Goldman and Sanjib K. Mukherjee

A Marketing Approach to Physician Recruitment by James Hacker, Don C. Dodson, and M. Thane Forthman

Marketing for CPAs, Accountants, and Tax Professionals edited by William J. Winston

Strategic Planning for Not-for-Profit Organizations by R. Henry Migliore, Robert E. Stevens, and David L. Loudon

Marketing Planning in a Total Quality Environment by Robert E. Linneman and John L. Stanton, Jr.

Managing Sales Professionals: The Reality of Profitability by Joseph P. Vaccaro

Squeezing a New Service into a Crowded Market by Dennis J. Cahill

Publicity for Mental Health Clinicians: Using TV, Radio, and Print Media to Enhance Your Public Image by Douglas H. Ruben

Managing a Public Relations Firm for Growth and Profit by A. C. Croft

Utilizing the Strategic Marketing Organization: The Modernization of the Marketing Mindset by Joseph P. Stanco

Internal Marketing: Your Company's Next Stage of Growth by Dennis J. Cahill

The Clinician's Guide to Managed Behavioral Care by Norman Winegar

Marketing Health Care into the Twenty-First Century: The Changing Dynamic by Alan K. Vitberg

Fundamentals of Strategic Planning for Health-Care Organizations edited by Stan Williamson, Robert Stevens, David Loudon, and R. Henry Migliore

Risky Business: Managing Violence in the Workplace by Lynne Falkin McClure

Predicting Successful Hospital Mergers and Acquisitions: A Financial and Marketing Analytical Tool by David P. Angrisani and Robert L. Goldman

Marketing Research That Pays Off: Case Histories of Marketing Research Leading to Success in the Marketplace edited by Larry Percy

How Consumers Pick a Hotel: Strategic Segmentation and Target Marketing by Dennis Cahill

Applying Telecommunications and Technology from a Global Business Perspective by Jay Zajas and Olive Church

Strategic Planning for Private Higher Education by Carle M. Hunt, Kenneth W. Oosting, Robert Stevens, David Loudon, and R. Henry Migliore

Writing for Money in Mental Health by Douglas H. Ruben

Writing for Money in Mental Health

Douglas H. Ruben, PhD

The Haworth Press
New York • London

The Haworth Press, Inc., 10 Alice Street, Binghamton, NY 13904-1580

Cover design by Marylouise E. Doyle.

Library of Congress Cataloging-in-Publication Data

Ruben, Douglas H.
    Writing for money in mental health / Douglas H. Ruben.
        p.   cm.
    Includes bibliographical references and index.
    ISBN 0-7890-0240-X (alk. paper).
    1. Mental health literature–Marketing. 2. Mental health literature–Publishing. 3. Mental health–Authorship. 4. Psychotherapy–Authorship. I. Title.
RC437.2.R83 1997
808′.066362–dc21

96-51806
CIP

CONTENTS

ABOUT THE AUTHOR

Douglas H. Ruben, PhD, is a clinical psychologist turned media specialist. He has a private practice but spends most of his time consulting authors, producers, literary agents, and publishers on book ideas and promotions. Dr. Ruben is the author or co-author of more than 34 books and 100 professional articles, ranging from scholarly to mass media self-helpers. His recent releases include *No More Guilt: 10 Steps to a Shame-Free Life; Bratbusters: Say Goodbye to Tantrums and Disobedience; Avoidance Syndrome: Doing Things Out of Fear; Family Recovery Companion; 60 Seconds to Success; One Minute Secrets to Feeling Great;* and *Publicity for Mental Health Clinicians* (The Haworth Press, Inc., 1995). Dr. Ruben's seminars on publishing and the media tour nationally and he regularly appears on TV and radio talk shows, including a recent appearance on *Donahue.*

Preface:
Turning Your Ideas into Dollars

My wife absolutely thinks I'm crazy because I have a crazy habit: I can't throw away old manuscripts. Manuscripts I wrote several years ago or even recently that never got published sit on a shelf and collect dust. They take up valuable space–like where a picture of the family or grandmother should sit–crammed into tiny spaces and dog-eared. I just can't throw them out. Of course, I know I should. But "what if," I ask myself, "What if I can revise these retired papers with the right magic to get them published?"

This sounds weird, doesn't it? Truth is, it's possible. I hate to toss out a manuscript if there's even the slightest chance of reviving it. I can breathe new air into a dying paper by altering its writing style.

Once upon a dinosaur time, when the manuscript was submitted to editors and rejected, reasons were a dime a dozen: "No thank you–it's not what we want," or "The writing style was different from our regular guidelines." My favorite was the "out-of-sync" reason: "Great idea," they would say, but wouldn't you know, "another article on the same topic has been accepted by us." Editors just accepted it one hour before my paper arrived. Bad Karma, I guess.

Probably. Luck has everything to do with the publishing field. Good luck is submitting a book or article when readers are famished for that topic. Write a book on domestic assault and submit it two days after O.J. Simpson's arrest, and you're in luck. Or how about if you submit a how-to book on teaching safety tips for opening suspicious-looking postal packages? Wouldn't you know it? Editors read it just as the FBI announces charges against the Unibomber. Now, that's lucky.

For most of us unlucky ones, however, timing is a matter of coincidence, unless, of course, you frequently win the lottery or have a special gift for astrology. Few of us claim this inherent fortune and must resort to the precise game of calibration. You have to plan, prioritize, and project the best time for a submission, trying to match it with newsworthy events. Fine-tuning that slippery dial between consumer need and your supply is a masterful art. Success only occurs when you can rapidly pump out proposals before headline stories become stale.

When it works, it's harmony. When it doesn't, your idea is garbage and you build a larger and larger stack of manuscripts on the shelf (what I call "paper death row"). Yes, one day these precious, well-considered, creative pieces will end up either as foodstuff for recycled paper or at the bottom of some landfill rotting away into oblivion.

That's probably why I have this habit: once I look at these death-row papers, I act as governor and give them amnesty. It's simply a shame to waste so much constructive thought without first retooling the idea, rewriting the paper, and seeking a new publishing route for it. While the downside is that my anal retentiveness keeps my office junked up, the upside is highly rewarding: Otherwise forgotten papers, into which much time, energy, and insight were invested can now reach a public. All that's needed is a smart marketing twist. Find an angle and pique an editor with it, and watch your good ideas be read. I've done it several times and know you'll have the joy of doing it yourself.

That's what this book is about. Somewhere in your house–in the basement, on the top shelf in a closet, even tucked away in boxes hiding underneath furniture–you have valuable, insightful ideas recorded on paper. It may be a thesis, dissertation, or even handouts you created when you taught college classes–all of these are expressions of your introspective mind. Now comes the grave-digging task of unearthing these lost papers and really asking yourself an honest question: "Can I save this thing?"

There's only one answer: "Yes." *Writing for Money in Mental Health* implores you to unwrap the mummified documents of ancient graduate days and your early professional career and revisit them with a refreshing new perspective. You can rejuvenate your ideas by using new tools to make these documents salable. Of course, if you are tired of these documents and more willing to let go than myself, go ahead—throw them out. You may handle separation better than I do. Nobody says *you have to resurrect these papers from the dead.* This is only one approach.

Another approach is to start from scratch. This means writing something brand new. Sounds impossible, doesn't it? First off, when do you have time to write it? During what hours of the day? While you're sleeping? How about between Sunday midnight and Monday morning, a period of time I refer to as "S'Monday." Finding unfilled hours in your day for creative writing may seem unlikely. You're probably exhausted just thinking of composing an article let alone a book. A *book*? Who has time in between seeing patients, billing third-party payers and, oh, yes, playing spouse and parent, to quietly seclude oneself for hours of typing? Do I look like David Thoreau? Does my busy lifestyle even come close to the peaceful utopia of *Walden*? Well, when you put it that way, I guess it probably doesn't.

Serious writers who publish for money are neither Henry David Thoreau nor, like Ernest Hemingway, do they retreat to summer homes on the ocean for relaxed writing. They are just like you and me. Their incredibly busy schedules and fast-paced routines stretch the 24-hour clock to its ultimate limits. They live the same life you live, except for one difference: ideas for books and articles pop into their minds during the day and they act on them either by constructing a proposal or seizing a canceled patient hour to type a few paragraphs.

Think of it this way: How many times have you sat in your office chair waiting for a late patient to arrive? There you are, with nothing to do, feeling unable to really begin a new task. After all, why begin something if you're only going to be interrupted when the patient shows up? That's the special reflective time you use to stare out the window or at your schedule book while entertaining many possibilities of what this world needs (for example, "What we need is a book on how to make patients punctual, or how about a patient's etiquette manual on seeking therapy!").

At other times, faced with extremely dysfunctional patients, your mind is an analytical engine. You're quick on your feet with amazing logical reasoning that combines theory with impeccable insight regarding some pathology. You suddenly stumble on a perfect cure or a remarkably lucid interpretation right in the middle of therapy. And, as timing would have it, your patient may even have blurted out, "Doctor So and So, you ought to write an article on that." What a coincidence. And you know why? They're right; you ought to write it.

That's what professional writers do. They seize an idea and follow it from start to finish before it vanishes from mind. The process of writing and inevitably selling your manuscript for money is not as difficult as it seems. All it takes is following simple rules of the trade. Sure, you need to have those *gestalt* moments of insight we spoke about a moment ago, but you have them all the time. Your training, experience, and clever ability to perceive phenomena from patient treatment put you way ahead of journalists who have to slave to interview people for this insight. You only need to interview your own brain—that's the easy part.

What may be scary is converting your mental pot of gold into a dynamite article or book. You're halfway there the moment you say, "If other people can do this, so can I." For every 100 self-help books riding a two-week shelf life, there is room on that shelf for another eye-catching book on the same subject. Even on subjects seemingly oversaturated with books (for example, sex and romance or parenting), the marketplace still demands newer, more appealing variations and is willing to pay big bucks for the next Jim Carrey of books.

Writing for Money in Mental Health will help you to realize your inner strengths in writing by showing you how you can take ideas and transform them into potential dollars using a variety of media. Today's advancing technology in computers, CDs, and the internet blasts open amazing opportunities for publishing in ways previously unimaginable. With a modem and a little ingenuity, your publishing outlets are practically infinite. Even if multimedia computers and cyberspace surfing are not your speed, a solid need remains for empirical, nonfiction articles and books in the commercial market. From quizzes and checklists on how to choose the right date to advice columns, pop magazines (*Good Housekeeping, Seventeen, Mademoiselle*) are starving animals waiting to feast on your spectacular thoughts. And that's not all. In the jungle of hungry sales merchants there are book publishers, software publishers, and TV and infomercial producers who don't want a small piece of the action; they want to corner the marketplace and are constantly on the lookout for fascinating, consumer-driven properties. Who says your next idea can't be fashioned to satisfy their appetite? The truth is that it can.

Writing for Money in Mental Health does more than just tell you how to sell your precious properties. It goes beyond what its predecessor *Publicity for Mental Health Clinicians* did. That book invited you to be a public relations agent in broadcasting your talents across the media airwaves and included your role in publishing. Now you can have updated information on traditional (magazine and book) publishing and get a leaping start on high-tech avenues for publishing and circulation. Even more, this book is tailored for mental health writers in the nonfiction marketplace and gives you specific lists of contacts. You can pinpoint the exact publisher, producer, or editor and know instantly what this person currently needs.

Having this database in one book hopefully will spare you the tedious research of investigating multiple lists for the general public that are not geared for your specialty. The time you will save from library digging is the time you can spend on developing a winning title, article, book, or proposal for the media frenzy.

Speaking of "frenzy," this reminds me of a second crazy habit I have. I tend to go like gangbusters on a writing project and at times forget what planet I live on. Those people who are dear to me and who interrupt my solitude to provide me with meals, remind me to sleep, and work to help support my endeavors. My wife, Marilyn, is a great example. She reminds me that there is a life beyond my computer; I'm glad I listen to her. Of course, now she's hooked on e-mail, multimedia computers, and is herself sequestered for hours in her own computer office. I guess it takes one to know one.

I also gratefully recognize the many generous contributors to this project who in one way or another furnished me with biographical information through e-mail, facsimile, or mail, or brought me articles and reprints during various stages of this book. Their support and enthusiasm tickled me with laughter and inspired the pages of this manual to be comprehensive while at the same time user-friendly. In particular, I wish to kindly thank Pamela Hodges for her insights on dogs and horses, and for informing me in her inimitable style that "Yes, there really are pet magazines that nonpet owners read." And, adding in her eloquent style, "C'mon, Doug, Akitas are always 100 pounds." Now I know that. Thanks, Pam.

Where writing for money really counts, I especially owe a debt of appreciation to my patients, friends, and relatives who have read, reread, and carefully commented on my self-help books and articles, offering me unusually acute perspectives on what today's commercial reader wants. They are my favorite audience, as I imagine your family and patients will be. All you need to do is undertake the exhilarating task of using your gifted talents and wisdom for well-earned, additional income.

PART I:
TIME FOR A CHANGE

Have you ever wondered about what motivates Olympic marathon runners? Is it their love of the outdoors? Maybe. How about the adrenaline-pumping rush they get from building up muscular endurance? Perhaps. What if the driving force for long-distance runners comes simply from the challenge; that is, can they actually outlast their opponents in an exhaustive, nearly debilitating exercise of mind over body? Now, that's a good question.

The same question can be asked of your own mind over body. For the average professional, daily tasks are all-consuming. Each day begins in high gear. You rush to take a sip of coffee and nibble a bagel for breakfast. (On bad days, it's only a power-bar.) Then you rush to fight traffic by car, bus, subway, or carpool in the nick of time for your first appointment. It doesn't matter where the destination is–clinic, hospital, nursing home, or private office–no sooner do you step inside the doorway then you're bombarded with unmerciful phone calls, e-mails, emergency paperwork, and meetings, all miserably interrupting the morning routines (that is, if there were routines).

Hospital and federal- or state-employed mental health providers run a rat race of urgently responding to some unfinished business. Usually, the unfinished business is someone else's. Days whisk by so quickly and often so unproductively that by evening there is only time to recuperate both emotionally and physically before starting the whole thing over again. It's back to fighting havoc the next morning.

The private practitioner equally fights the traffic of life obstacles. In one- to two-person offices, unlike larger agencies, clerical support is minimal, and all clerical activities from report writing to billing to faxing are miraculously squeezed in between seeing clients. Open-hour slots get filled quickly returning phone calls. A mental health provider wears many hats: sometimes he or she is a clerk, other times a collections agent, and still other times a compassionate therapist.

Multiple priorities get juggled, and therapists stay calm and cool, or at least they try to; in fact, they can't afford not to. I'm reminded right now of the therapist who in a single hour talked a person out of suicide; helped a family with a violent child's behavior, which required psychiatric hospital admission; and somehow managed to return two new phone referrals. But here's the impressive part: come the next hour, the therapist smiled from ear to ear and enthusiastically greeted the next appointment. Now, that's quick recuperation of the zenith type.

The price tag for being busy is loneliness. Busy lives in both the private and public mental health sectors allow for few outside interests except for long-standing hobbies, family activities, and religious practices. Outside of these limited social parameters, today's providers are at a loss for how to create more hours in their already suffocating daily time schedules.

Efficient time management is not the only answer. There are only so many hours in the day. What will magically cure the exhausting roller coaster of tasks? Megavitamins? No. Intense aerobic workouts or daily weight lifting? Probably not. Nothing against bodybuilding, but such power strategies are no substitute for the real test of fortifying your mental ambition.

There are a variety of ways to rise above the rat race. You can achieve career growth, and with it salary growth, through promotion. However, years may pass before a job promotion is feasible. Supplementing and eventually doubling your income by writing is an easier passage to financial success. While you're slowly, but surely hiking up the executive ladder, dollars equivalent to years of promotions can be earned fast.

You may already be a writer. Chances are you have been an author, editor, or compiler of several academic and trade paperback books; so, you read these pages thinking to yourself, "What's the big deal?"

I'll tell you what the big deal is. A prolific author doesn't make a rich author. Scores of scholars populate the prestigious academic journals in mental health specialties. Does that make these authors wealthy? Some authors, especially those of textbooks or measurement instruments and tests that evolved into subsequent editions, updated versions, and translations into multiple languages are quite wealthy. The percentage of royalty-wealthy scholarly and reference-writing authors, however, is miserably low.

You can amass 20 books that are all ideally suited for graduate reading and sold to college libraries. It's a real high going into any college library and typing your name into the computer search code. You discover your name and all of your books referenced there. It's great fun—whoopee—but you didn't earn much money on them.

That's when a sad realization hits you like a ton of bricks: scholarly books don't pay—not 20 of them, not 30 of them, not even 40 of them. So, just being an author is not enough.

An author who sells his or her work either by receiving advances or outright purchases is a prolific writer in a different way. That author makes money doing it. Productivity is higher when the underlying incentive for writing is dollars and cents. When you accept an advance of $2,000 for a ghostwriting assignment, for example, and are promised additional dollars paid upon completion of the next installment, guess what happens? You definitely feel an urge to write.

This section underscores the basic tenet that writing for money is a mind-building and financially healthy venture that can be incorporated into your life in less time than you think. Composing original pieces that somebody will pay you a respectable fee for begins with knowing how much you can charge and realistically how much you can receive. These next two chapters will introduce the fundamentals of undertaking this enterprise and hopefully whet your appetite.

Chapter 1

Short on Cash?

Today's high-octane, high-action lifestyle puts enormous pressure on pushing yourself above and beyond your personal limitations. Think of it: extra hours worked on weekends; responses to emergency patients calling late at night; and rushing to write, type or send in reports. Sounds crushing, doesn't it? And the writing part of your job is incessant. Since managed-care systems took over, report writing is a daily diet that produces extensive patient progress reports and requests for session authorizations. In all, practitioners probably spend more time in front of their PCs than in front of deeply needy patients.

As freedom from the "paper-prison" vanishes, so does the income generated from clinical practice. Salaries qouted in the last decade under nonmanaged private practice were significantly higher than today's deflated earnings. This is due to cost-containment policies of session limits and diverting patient referrals to in-house clinicians rather than to contract or "outside" providers (Doverspike, 1995; Goodman, Brown, and Deitz, 1992). Diminished revenues of 20 to 30 percent, largely blamed on premiums for rapid-treatment closures, have cost independent practitioners from $10,000 to $15,000 in lost income over a two-year period. Similar wage losses are attributed to patients with third-party payers that offer lower reimbursements per session to nonparticipating providers than to their participating providers (Ruben and Stout, 1983; Spitz, 1996; Stout, 1996).

The results have been dismal for financially struggling therapists. Many have gone out of business affiliated themselves with established outpatient clinical agencies. Some have accepted work for hospitals and government agencies only to have discovered unforgivable constraints on their autonomy and to have suffered plunging wages. The upside has been freedom from "hitting the pavement" for new referrals and billing headaches, as well as reliable clerical support and centralized accounting departments to administer billing and collect unpaid debts.

However, what they gained in credit and referral-building relief, they lost in terms of advancing potential for higher salary and distinction. Base salaries at state and federal levels are minimally $50,000 to $60,000 lower than the average annual earning of a full-time private practitioner. Those who are under contract with another agency are equally gouged by percentages paid to the "house." Most clinics want between 40 to 50 percent of dollars earned per patient session in return for providing office space and clerical services.

This jaw-dropping reality slowly paced its way throughout the nation, affecting only a handful of part-time therapists. Now, with more graduating therapists vying for patient referrals, and with increased competition between HMOs, PPOs, and psychology managed-care groups, larger majorities of full-time providers feel the economic hardships of paycheck cuts (Gumpert, 1995). They are unhappy, deeply worried, and are finally realizing that survival in the therapist marketplace may require generating income from less traditional resources.

That is what this chapter addresses. Shortage of treatment income necessitates a creative alternative to covering overhead costs and restoring the lifestyle to which most providers have grown accustomed. Yes, there are therapists reportedly comfortable with their incomes and perhaps even insulated from national trends in managed care, but they, too, recognize that a stable income may not last forever and that prudence dictates having a back-up plan in case the flow of cash suddenly stops.

First, let's briefly consider the most common entrepreneurial ways therapists have produced income, followed by several "not-so-common" ways. From there, we will review even "strange" ways of diving into the "sea of green." At the end, I will present a hard-copy look at exactly what the current market pays for different variations of writing, whether it be for books, magazines, or electronic media. Needless to say, once your eyes stare at the impressively high-dollar figures earnable in writing, you may wonder why it took you so long to wipe the dust off your computer.

COMMON WAYS OF EARNING EXTRA DOLLARS

The infinitely large number of ways money is earned can hardly be explored within one book. Scores of successfully wealthy individuals made their fortunes through sales, the stock market, industrial products, sports, or by Hollywood fame. Winners of the lottery, royalty, and beneficiaries of inheritances may live in the lap of luxury, but they are not really engineers of hard-earned income.

In the mental health field, frequently providers are ingeniously productive in finding alternative sources of revenue. Some take on extra jobs in hopes of supplementing income and expanding their referral bases. Others who are more adventurous invent new methods or products directly marketed to their target consumers—sometimes patients, sometimes the general public—through whom they hope to expand other product lines. Together these money-making ideas account for the following common ventures.

Teaching

Centuries of scholarly tradition in universities and community colleges is proof that mental health practitioners have a home in teaching. Today's doctoral graduates in science-practitioner models and purely practitioner models are inculcated from their first core class to become academics. This naturally opens the door for full-time providers to be part-time instructors or for full-time instructors to be part-time providers.

The downside of teaching is purely economic. Compensation for full-semester (or quarter) classroom instruction is peanuts compared to patient session fees. One can literally generate enough money in one week of therapy to equal an instructor's pay for a 15-week semester. And, at least in my estimate, your time is worth many more dollars earned through other rewarding occupations.

Testing

An usual adjunct to clinical practice is testing. Most therapists trained and licensed to administer tests will maximize this component for additional revenue. Testing offers lucrative advantages if marketed correctly, prepared accurately, and when it serves a needed population. For example, neuropsychological testing batteries in theory last ten hours and run between $2,000 to $5,000 for the complete diagnostic. That's a lot of money.

For any clinician able to truly collect this fee on a regular basis, I personally bow to their unprecedented success. However, few agencies, managed care groups, or patients are willing to hand over such an incredible amount of cash no matter how prestigious the examiner or impressive the results. Plan on being paid a disappointing $300 to $500 for two to four hours of an abbreviated battery. Even in forensic examination—that is, where testing is done on competency to stand trial or for child-custody cases—compensation is still meager because it is not calculated based on the provider's expertise.

Testing generates a poor return unless one does a lot of testing or has worked out a deal with an agency or managed-care group as sole examiner for particular diagnostic problems.

Moonlighting

When one day job doesn't quite pay expenses, a second therapy job after work hours is pursued. Providers committed to a standard nine-to-five business day find they can explore their clinical roots and see private patients from 5 p.m. to 9 p.m., thereby enjoying extra income without interfering with their day job. On the surface, this is a sound idea for budget-squeezers, going from paycheck to paycheck and supporting a family.

Still, moonlighting has a dark side. It is very tiring. Fatigue is by far the dominant reason why after-work therapists give up on clinical work. They instantly realize that after a long workday their mind and body lack the stamina and perceptual energy needed to keenly assess and treat demanding patients. The few extra dollars profited from a week's worth of overtime simply doesn't justify feeling like roadkill by the weekend.

Consulting

Practitioners are experts by design. They already possess a highly complex repertoire of knowledge on so many aspects of human behavior that translating this knowledge into a consulting role is effortless. Consulting for most therapists is on therapy. They may give workshops, talks, seminars, keynote addresses, or even oversee projects as specialists. In forensic work, consulting pays a higher purse when one acts as an expert witness in a deposition or courtroom, or if asked by the prosecution, defense, or police force for input in their steps of discovery.

Forensic consulting pays from $250 to $1,000 per hour, depending on your experience, expertise, and reputation among attorneys. Say, for example, you superbly deciphered the handwriting of a suspect in a murder trial, which led to a conviction. Rumor of your commanding success as a "behavioral profiler" will rapidly circulate through the legal grapevine and bring you other jobs.

But forensic work has its serious pitfalls. As with any high-paying job, the risks are also high. Courtroom appearances are meat markets where the prosecuting and defense attorneys are carnivores who have every legal right to slice and dice up your replies, your personality, and your academic training in hopes of discrediting your testimony. That's their job. That's what they were trained to do. With so much riding on your credibility each time you enter the courtroom, few mental health practitioners want to stick their neck out for the bucks. They decide not to make a living in forensics.

Supervising

Now here is a prosperous market. Three decades ago, the role of supervisor was a privileged status where a seasoned, talented mentor could truly sculpt the paths of freshman in mental health. It was an honor studying under prestigious mentors who had published and had community notoriety.

That was then. Today the image of a supervisor has drastically been defaced as an avaricious and manipulating person whose primary concerns are control and authority. Now, that doesn't mean all supervisors are bad apples. Not all supervisors take fiscal and emotional advantage over their subordinates, and plenty of them are still as honorable as their predecessors. But most money earned from supervision is largely the result of state licensing rules not only in psychology but also in counseling, rehabilitation, and in many factions therein (e.g., nurse practitioners). These rules absolutely demand residency or internships for several months up to two years. So, for a length of time, many therapists are at the mercy of paying supervisors exorbitant fees to continue their livelihood.

Fees charged for supervision run the scale from top to bottom. Per-hour fees start as low as $40 and jump off the map at $150–all defended as a necessary stage in a student's learning process. While this appears to be a profitable enterprise, ask yourself if the glamour is short-lived. Supervisors, no matter what they charge, are intimately responsible for the professional conduct of their subordinates. Should, for example, a supervised therapist engage in sexual relations with a patient, this egregiously unethical behavior and any resulting litigation is jointly shared between therapist and supervisor. Neither are spared the humiliating and ultimately costly legal fees accrued in the case. Along with the responsibility of monitoring the student's interventions, there is also a legal obligation to ensure that students behave as professionals.

Grants and Projects

Experimental psychologists have long been aware of research opportunities through funded grants. Limited and long-term grants are awarded by both the government and private foundations, who actively seek and receive proposals for inspiring projects ranging from animal drug studies to substance abuse therapies. Governmental grants, for example, from the National Institute of Mental Health (NIMH) or subdivisions within that branch (bureaus on aging, alcohol and drug abuse, etc.) generously donate unconditional funds to published researchers whom the agency trusts will produce valuable results.

"Unconditional" means that the money is not paid back at some later date. In return for generous funds, which go toward paying individual salaries as well as purchasing supplies, research results become the exclusive, legal property of the donor.

Naturally, financially insightful practitioners view grants with great fondness. They automatically believe that a good project deserves funding and will be a guaranteed salary for a year or two. But stop the presses; there's news they have not heard yet. Grants are *extremely difficult to get.* Remember those statistics on being struck by lightening? Or the odds you'd have to beat to win the lottery? Well, being awarded a grant is not that far off in improbability.

The reason grants are unreliable goldmines is twofold. First, writing a grant is extremely arduous, meticulous, and redundant. You must explain to death the benefits versus risks valued on the subjects under study. Second, the steps you must take even before you actually take the plunge to grant writing are enormous. The biggest one is called politicking. If you have friends in high places—in this case Washington, DC—then no problem. Or, if your clinic, agency, or school is already a grant recipient due for renewal, no problem. Or, if you're a nonprofit organization, your chances are strong.

But watch out if you're Mr. Nobody. Candidates are subject to ethics review approval, they must have impeccable credentials, and they must be able to pay lip service to the funding committee and provide every additional piece of paper that is requested. Sure, it's "do-able," but who has time, right?

Well, many do. There are veteran grant writers and recipients who literally subsist on one grant following another grant. They are to be commended, since the rest of us would find the process deeply upsetting and a waste of time.

UNCOMMON WAYS OF EARNING EXTRA DOLLARS

Off the beaten track from conventional dollar-raising activities are some other ambitious endeavors undertaken by only a minority of practitioners. Few actually delve into this murky terrain because of the technical or political jockeying that goes on in the process. While practitioners are skillful enough, skill is only one-half of the equation. It takes time, effort, and energy after a long patient-seeing day to re-energize oneself for extra activities. As you will see, many of the uncommon ways may strike you as "common" ways since your colleagues already engage in these activities. So, consider as you read these why you, yourself, don't do them.

Writing Books

Authoring your ideas in a book is a brilliant expression of personal integrity, insight, and clinical experience. It articulately spells out your position on theories, methods, and case studies with literary license for you to be imaginative in your presentation. Whether in medical or mental health, practitioners-turned-writers magnetically are drawn to writing certain books because they know what their patients like and what they will buy (Dunn and Hansen, 1995). And those are the best insider's tips on marketing one could ever have.

McCollough (1994) got right to the point, when she said that people buy books because the author is an expert. She's right: authors are professional authorities who carry incredible clout among this country's book buyers. Combine this venerable voice with a strong self-help theme and publishers will scramble over each other like mice to offer that authority a contract.

Since definitions of self-help are so broad, topics on any subject are in open season. Starker (1989) was among the first to recognize this phenomenon. The outpouring of diet, exercise, and success books written by health care professionals doubled in a decade and could not entirely satisfy the consumer's feeding frenzy. Each chapter prescribing a new strategy, belief, or religion captured the wounded hearts of recovery-book readers looking for that one solution to their nagging problems. When they found it, not only did they munch on the book they bought, but in a panic rage of bingeing, gobbled up all other books either written by the same author or on the same subject. Such a consumer following has been evident for Wayne Dwyer and Claudia Black, among others. They are gurus in their area because a faithful, dollar-paying public demands their products.

So, why don't more practitioners write books? The first book in this series (Ruben, 1995) addressed that issue. Health practitioners are fearful of submitting their ideas in print in front of editors or peer reviewers who may—and usually do—reject the manuscript. To vulnerably expose trade secrets for an editor to make harsh marks with a red pen is a bit too nauseating for most providers. It freaks them out, and I agree; it hurts. But it hurts going through a doctoral program, and many mental health providers did that.

Fear stands in the way if the mechanics of writing and reaching publishers are unknown. Once they are known, things suddenly change. The anxiety disappears and would-be writers embark on scribing marathons until they at least have a chapter to send out.

Writing Magazine Articles and Newspaper Columns

Stretch your imagination even farther, and picture a glossy black-and-white photo of yourself beaming from newsprint alongside your column. Newspaper and magazine writing is a common money-making option. Contributors submit weekly articles of one to three pages on some contemporary or newsworthy issue, or have a column dedicated to responding to letters sent in by readers, and get a byline naming who they are.

Some magazine writers take this writing magic a step further by preparing a longer or "feature" article running 5 to 10 pages or about 2,500 to 5,000 words. They try to publish it in commercial magazines such as *People, Glamour, GQ,* and *House and Garden.* Editors are willing to send submission guidelines to help writers know how to write their articles and to inform them about what currently is in vogue for their magazines.

And payment? Well, we'll get to that later. Needless to say, payment upon acceptance can range from $25 to $5,000 depending on the topic, whether or not it contains an interview, and the reputation of the author. Got an interview with David Duchorny, star celebrity of the hit thriller *X-Files*? That will generate a proud fee of $4,000 in many upscale commercial magazines.

With dollars just waiting to be paid for magazine writing, why aren't mental health providers biting the bait? Again, it's that "time and fear thing." Overcoming the trembling fear that somebody may actually read your ideas is one thing; putting these ideas down in print and sending them off to a magazine is another.

The other downside is competition. Without insider tips, writing for magazines can be a lost cause. Busy editors who receive over-the-transom submissions—that is, unsolicited manuscripts—may dump these at the bottom of the slush pile. When they actually get reviewed, you will probably be somewhere between your seventieth and eightieth birthdays. But calling ahead, pitching your story directly to the acquisitions editor, or even sending a flash fax will alert the editor that you mean business. And if you got their attention in one way, confidence is built; they know you will get the attention of their readers.

Media Consulting

More and more of today's motion pictures and TV movies have violent themes or are about child and spouse abuse. As new factually based dramas overlap with psychological themes, mental health specialists have suddenly become a vital commodity for movie producers. In *Publicity for Mental Health Clinicians* (1995), chapters 11 and 12 entirely address how this parade of jobs is growing exponentially and can be a versatile avocation for mental health providers.

Bouhoutsos (1990) is also a big advocate of media psychology. She sees psychologists, social workers, and allied health practitioners as forerunners in educating the public and perfect for the role of communicators. Her voice represents a loud voice in Division 26 of the American Psychological Association on Media Psychology, which effectively promotes an open invitation for health professionals to enter the airwaves.

So, why don't more people join the bandwagon and appear on the eleven o'clock news? Sure, blame it on being scared. Fear is the catch-all for all of our failures. But this time, fear takes a second row seat. There's a stronger reason: therapists don't know how to get started. Once a relationship is established between the therapist and a station's news director or a producer, the rest is a piece of cake. But it takes time to learn the ropes of the trade. Where to start, how to get there, and what to do when the opportunity smacks you in the face at first are mysteries until somebody teaches you these things. They are obstacles producing heavy avoidance.

Managed Care Consulting

Still another endeavor recently popping up in the mental health jobline is helping organizations design and implement psychiatry managed-care programs. This task involves experienced financial officers or those with a solid background in running managed-care systems. Consultants turn to the public sector for hired services.

They offer skillful direction, troubleshooting tips, and in effect hold the agency's hand through each step of engineering the program. Consulting fees are around $150 to $300 per hour depending on experience, savvy, and credentials. Clearly, this pathway is a riveting new venture for entrepreneurial-minded professionals able to sell themselves.

And that's where the buck stops. Because this source of consulting is in demand, bidders must be salespeople. They must outdo the caliber of competition by being versatile and putting on a "dog and pony show." But who likes to sell? Selling is a turnoff for many providers who are conservative. They believe their name and services, much like physicians, will naturally gain the respect of the community and in turn lead to referrals. For many, that's exactly what happens. Overdosing the marketplace, some feel, with posterboard ads on "why I'm so great . . . and you're not" seems pretentious, arrogant, and simply not professional.

That is why there are those who survive clinical practice and those who do not. The survivors make exceptions to this unwritten "no advertising rule" by creatively stimulating consumer interest. Those who close up shop maintain their moral scruples but do not have a practice to help people the way they were trained to do.

STRANGE WAYS OF EARNING EXTRA DOLLARS

Money-making vehicles for staying afloat in rough economic seas are plentiful. Many mental health providers already realize this and are thoroughly reaping the financial benefits from their activities. With a little courage, training, and know-how (and don't forget luck), adventures down the prosperous brick road are not elusive and can be easy ways to supplement a clinical practice.

Faced with a drop in caseload and a dry spell in referrals, therapists have been forced to dig down into their treasure chests of ideas or borrow from other professions to pay the monthly rent. None of these creative undertakings are illegal, unethical, or even slightly unbecoming of a practitioner; they are just not commonly associated with your run-of-the-mill therapist. That is why I list them here and will expand upon them in the course of this book.

Ghostwriting and Editing

For years, consultants offering to repair, spruce up, and do surgery on your written words enjoyed a thriving business in the fiction and nonfiction writers' market. One glance through the classifieds of periodicals such as *The Writer, Writer's Digest,* and other trade magazines revealed the multiplicity of one-stop editorial "stores" whose services specialized in helping you reach your goal.

And what is that goal? Well, certainly Scarecrow, it is "to get a brain."

The consultant associated with any such "store" acts as the brainchild to rewrite your text so that it magnetically draws publishers' attention. Editors who do this job are called "scriptdoctors." Scriptdoctors either can take what you have and revise it, or they can turn your ideas into a magazine or book. In that way, scriptdoctors take no credit as author, but as *ghostwriter.* More and more mental health providers, confident in their writing, are advertising themselves as ghostwriters and editors for the extra money.

How much money? Well, think of it this way: for an average edited manuscript of 400 pages, charged at $3.50 per page, the total is $1,400. That's for reading and rewriting a book, and it's pretty easy once you know how. Prices go higher when credentials show you're not only a whiz at polishing up words, but also when your finished product impresses a publisher at first glance and the author gets a publishing contract. Now, you're cooking!

Ghostwriting is a different animal altogether. Fees vary, with some ghostwriters setting a flat fee, paid in installments during the writing of the book, and others taking a huge chunk of the royalties if they honestly believe the book is dynamite or when the book idea is under publisher contract. Still other ghostwriters charge on an hourly basis. Contracts may pay anywhere from $5,000 to $20,000 for writing another person's book, and your name may never appear anywhere on the manuscript.

Ghostwriting is very different from scholarly writing. Codes of authorship in research and scholarly publications require all significant contributors to be named as authors and less significant "helpers" to be thanked in acknowledgments. This is what confused me when I began ghostwriting. For instance, I felt a sudden urge to beg the author for my name to appear alongside his or her name, thinking this was the "right thing to do."

Smartly, I remembered that the right thing to do was to remain silent. These kind authors paid me dearly to remain invisible and make only themselves look good. It's a humbling experience to have your name left off a manuscript that you wrote. You learn to swallow your pride in the interest of serving other people—a lesson from which a good practitioner can benefit.

Scriptwriting

When you have a sudden insight into what people should learn or what skills may benefit employees, you've got the stuff of which corporate scriptwriting is made. Scriptwriting can involve writing for the movies, perhaps even big-screen motion pictures. For this book, however, scriptwriting only deals with writing industrial and corporate videos, TV infomercials, and some other TV projects. Fashioning yourself as a Hollywood screenwriter, in other words, is not the image hoped for here. Yes, it certainly can happen, and there are many counselors turned scriptwriters and scriptwriters turned "psyche-writers" who could convincingly sell you on how to make it to the top. Ask scripter Steve Levitt, for example. He's a happy camper these days. On only a verbal pitch—no title, no written words—his psychological story of a gay Harvard professor adopting a stripper's baby earned $250,000 in advanced royalties against $500,000 paid in total from Turner pictures.

Don't go auctioning your practice just yet. Screenwriting is *very, very* tough and very frustrating. The main reason for this is simple: *You must know somebody to do anything in the business. Or, if you do it yourself . . . it takes lots of money.*

Scripting corporate and infomercial television is acting as surgeon for an existing script. Corliss (1994) remarked that screenplays are frequently rewritten at the last moment, often overlooking the scriptdoctor who responded to the producer's 911 call. Uncredited scriptdoctors such as Robert Towne, whose revisions included *Bonnie and Clyde* and *The Godfather,* live a secret life except when called in urgently during the middle of production. What they lack in bylines they make up in salaries. Supplemental incomes for scriptdoctors of screenplays range from $60,000 to $100,000.

When screen or TV credit is given, watch how your career can skyrocket into orbit. Joss Whedon, an unknown yesterday, for example, jumped to number one on the billboard after he did radical surgery on Kevin Costner's aqua-picture *Waterworld*. While Costner's ocean drama film sunk, Whedon's career tidal-waved. His other retooling effort was for a box-office hit *Speed*.

Acting as Literary Agent

Experienced authors and newcomers alike are taking the business into their own hands. Rather than entrust an intermediary to represent their best interests to publishers, authors are eagerly reversing the process and having publishers not only call them, but acting as their own agents. Agents traditionally are the negotiators, the schmoozers, and sell the publisher on buying your book. Because agents have for many years been the only gatekeeper to publishers, authors were forced to use their services. Manipulative agents thrived on this monopoly. They selectively promoted authors who they felt had a chance and who generated revenue for the agent, while downplaying and ignoring unknowns. The truth came out eventually, however. After a while, unknown authors got the message and found that it was not their manuscript that was weak but the agent's contacts who only wanted certain market guarantees. That's when the tables turned.

Today, more and more publishers have an open-door policy, inviting unpublished authors to call and discuss their proposals. Authors call, hear what publishers have to say, and even negotiate contracts over the phone. One can polish the "do-it-yourself" approach fairly quickly and eventually reach a point where he or she can help out another author. That's what makes you an effective negotiator-agent for a colleague. You are clearly more sympathetic to a peer's book and have the sensitivity to explain the ups and downs in language your peer will understand and deeply appreciate.

Agents get paid one of two ways: they either enjoy an up-front fee or receive a hefty percentage of the royalty.

Constructing a Web Page

It is no surprise that computer technology is light years from where it was a decade ago. We can "surf" to the outer limits. Some readers of this book may remember their undergraduate years struggling with mainframe computers and wondering if there was ever an end in sight. Well, there was. It happened in 1978 with the advent of microchip computers. And that was the beginning of the computer revolution.

Now computers act as telephones enabling modem connections to worldwide receivers. This phenomenal outreach, which begins at your fingertips and ends thousands upon thousands of miles across the globe, is called the *Internet*. This magnificent forum for correspondence has been an educational godsend for uploading and downloading huge masses of valuable information. That's why advertisers want a piece of the action. Where there are people, there will be a system of economy. Advertisers want to sell things and people want to buy things. Sold on the internet are a multitude of products from toys to games to videos to services to deals with oil refineries. Any and all products made artistically appealing and able to stand out in the morass of confusing cybernoise will win in the marketing war.

The device each advertiser uses for product publicity is a page on the *World Wide Web*. The web is a multimedia engine that whirls and twirls with sound, video, and three-dimensional graphics that illuminate a product to near virtual reality. But for every product wanting web site exposure, there must be a person who can construct that web site. And that is where many mental health providers who are artistic and computer literate are making money.

On-Line Therapy

Imagine the future in cyberspace: groceries bought on-line; entire academic programs run through e-mail and web sites; and real estate televideoed into your living room, where you can watch a three-dimensional tour of your prospective house. The truth is that many of these Star Trek innovations are actually in phases of development or already exist in some capacity.

The newest on-line vehicle for consumers is therapy. On-line psychological services are interactive systems whereby patients can talk via internet to an invisible therapist whose words of wisdom reply back in a bulletin-board-like fashion. Inspiring on-line therapy, obviously, is cheaper sessions and immediacy of therapist interaction. For example, check out a call-a-shrink website for panic anxiety (http://frank.mtsu.du/sward/anxiety.html).

A large constituency of curious mental health providers are seriously thinking of driving on the superhighway. They believe it holds enormous flexibility for time and cost and relieves them of office overhead expenses. Attractive, also, is the speed with which payments through major credit cards can eliminate tedious billing practices and the inevitable drag of collections.

Still, this constituency is one voice in a vast pool of skeptical onlookers. Even the American Psychological Association (APA) doesn't really know what to make of it. They are watching carefully and weighing the pros and cons before posturing a position. I don't blame them. While intuitively it seems that on-line therapy is not really therapy since basic dynamics of face-to-face counseling are absent, one cannot dismiss the benefits in responsivity of contact, affordability, and widespread use. More consumers than ever are flocking to their computer screens to hear what Doctor So and So has to say. These consumers definitely want psychological services, and as a result it is upscaling the image of therapy.

The formula is simple: *Market success is the living breath of any business,* and APA or other allied health organizations are probably going to put the verdict on hold until all the data are entirely in.

HOW MUCH ARE YOU WORTH?

Did you ever do a study of how many hours you actually spend a day or a week in your office? Twelve hours a day? Maybe 60 hours a week, give or take a lunch break here or there and including weekend spot checks or emergency calls? I would imagine these figures are right up your alley. Full-time practitioners are averaging 60 to 80 hours per week between patient sessions, paperwork, and marketing. They begin working early and stay late hours. At the end of their fiscal year, sizing up their annual salary, they can reflectively be proud of working so hard.

But is that salary really proportional to your effort? That is what we ask here and throughout the book, as the prospect of *writing for money* seizes your attention. Table 1.1 is your first temptation. It's a list of fascinating endeavors that will be covered in subsequent chapters, and provides recommended prices you can charge for different services or money you can expect to earn appear for each endeavor. Payments and fees will naturally vary by the provider's experience in the field, salesmanship, and geography. Fees in Manhattan, for example, drastically are higher than fees charged in Wyoming. These fees and payments draw from a sample of individuals nationwide who are currently providing these services. We will hear more about some of these in later chapters.

TABLE 1.1. Fees and payments for various writing endeavors

FOR WRITING A SELF-HELP BOOK

Advances: $500 to $4,000
Royalty given: 5% to 10%
Dollars earned/yr.: $500 to $2,000 (based on net sales of copies sold)

FOR WRITING A MAGAZINE ARTICLE

Payment on acceptance: $1.00 to $3.00/word
Number of words: 240 to 4,000 words

FOR SCRIPTING A CORPORATE VIDEO AND REWRITING SCRIPTS

Outright purchase for script: $300 to $4,000
Per minute price: $75 to $120 for one reel
Scripting for TV (teleplays): $5,000 to $14,000
Rewriting Scripts: $500 to $2,000

FOR SCRIPTING AN INFOMERCIAL

Outright purchase: $5,000 to $15,000
Hourly fee: $40 to $80/hour

FOR WRITING SOFTWARE (NOT PROGRAMMING IT)

Software manual (technical) writing: $30 to $50/hour
Software programs described, not written: $300 to $3,000
Royalty for software programs: 5% to 8%

FOR GHOSTWRITING AND EDITING

Book proposal writing: $200 to $3,500
Ghostwriting magazine for physician: $2,000 to $4,000
Magazine editing: $15 to $30/hour

TABLE 1.1 (continued)

Manuscript consultation: $25 to $50/hour
Consultant to publisher: $100 to $500 per book review
Ghostwriting book, total contract: $5,000 to $20,000
Ghostwriting book, per hour: $30 to $60/hour
Ghostwriting book, royalty percentage: 15% to 50%
Rewriting: $2.00 to $5.00/page
Submission package: $200 to $500

FOR ACTING AS LITERARY AGENT

Reading fees: $150 to $200*
Quarterly clerical fees: $75 to $100 (for clerical costs)
Royalty percentage on domestic sales: 10% to 20% of author's percentage
Royalty percentage on international/subsidy rights sales: 50% of author's percentage (which is usually split 50/50 with publisher)

FOR CONSTRUCTING A WEB PAGE

For simple one-page website: $250 to $500
For simple multiple page website (subsites): $450 to $1,500
For multimedia, multiple page website (subsites): $2,500 to $6,000

*Certain union laws forbid or strongly discourage upfront reading fees. For example, Writers Guild of America (WGA) signatories, that is, those agencies accepted into the WGA's roster who represent screenplays, are strictly prohibited from charging submission or reading fees. Book agents, while not governed by union guidelines, may charge moderate fees but are leaning toward free readings.

REFERENCES

Bouhoutsos, J.C. (1990). Media psychology and mediated therapeutic communication. In G. Gumpert and S.L. Fish (Eds.), *Talking to strangers: Mediated therapeutic communication. Communication and information science,* pp. 54-72. Norwood, NJ: Ablex Publishing.

Corliss, R. (1994). Miracle surgery: When a big movie like *Speed* or *Wolf* has an ailing screenplay, Hollywood calls in the script doctors. *Time,* July 25 (Vol. 44, No. 4) p. 60.

Doverspike, W. (1995). Some survival tips for dealing with insurance companies and managed care. In L. Vandercreek, S. Knapp, and T.L. Jackson (Eds.), *Innovations in clinical practice.* Sarasota, FL: Professional Resource Exchange.

Dunn, A.H. and Hansen, C.J. (1995). *Nonacademic writing: Social theory and technology.* Hillsdale, NJ: Lawrence Erlbaum Associates.

Goodman, M., Brown, J. and Deitz, P. (1992). *Managing managed care: A mental health practitioner's survival guide.* Washington, DC: American Psychiatric Press.

Gumpert, P. (1995). The therapist as dragonslayer: Confronting industrialized mental health. In M. Sussman (Ed.), *A perilous calling: The hazards of psychotherapy practice.* NY: John Wiley & Sons.

McCollough, V. E. (1994). Want to write for the lay press? Try a self-help angle. *American Medical News,* 37 (9), p. 50.

Ruben, D.H. (1995). *Publicity for mental health clinicians: Using TV, radio, and print media to enhance your public image.* Binghamton, NY: The Haworth Press, Inc.

Ruben, D.H. and Stout, C. (1983). *Transitions: Handbook of managed care for inpatient to outpatient treatment.* Westport, CT: Praeger Press.

Spitz, H.I. (1996). *Group psychotherapy and managed mental health care: A clinical guide for providers.* NY: Brunner/Mazel.

Starker, S. (1989). *Oracle at the supermarket: The American preoccupation with self-help books.* New Brunswick, NJ: Transaction Publishers.

Stout, C. (1996). *The complete guide to managed behavioral healthcare.* NY: John Wiley & Sons.

Chapter 2

One Hundred Bucks Says
You Can Self-Market

In the Sunday classifieds section of most daily newspapers are large display ads for used-car dealerships, furniture stores, and computer discount stores. The quarter-page, half-page, and full-page ads literally scream out to you with neon lights, and it's hard to miss their compelling messages: BUY ME!

Lured by what's written (the copy) you can't help but spot the words in bold print alongside a humorous graphic. "Clever," you might mutter to yourself, thinking that smart people created this advertisement. Although not in the market today for what they're selling, you know that if you were, that ad alone would drive you to a purchase. That's what marketing does. This chapter covers the basics on marketing your proposal to the right source. Steps on how to send materials and critical decision-making techniques keep your chances alive for a successful sale and placement of your manuscript.

Think of marketing this way: Product marketing is qualifying your special idea (in this case, a proposal) as a potential purchase by consumers. Who you identify as consumers will vary. Book and magazine proposals are for consumers who are publishers. Software proposals are either for publishers, producers, distributors, developers, or the general public. TV and video proposals and scripts are for producers. Targeting the right consumer is just as important as designing the methodology for that consumer.

Consumer selection also enables a closer inspection of what similar products already bombard the consumer. You need to know this because it determines how your product must be different. Products promising a strong improvement over competitive products and offering longer or permanent effects are more desirable and usually do better in sales (Braus, 1992).

This is where a technical strategy for self-marketing comes into play. You can write one, considering how "in-touch" you are with consumer needs. You, as self-marketer and therapist, already have your finger on the pulse of what your patients want. You know what they read and what applications and services they use on the computer. You are several steps ahead of journalists and non-mental-health providers who rely on guesswork, demographic statistics, or mailing lists. Inside your sessions or from field experience, you gain valuable leads on the "human stockmarket." This is because you are an active trader on the health care industry exchange (Starker, 1990).

You know when buying trends for certain merchandise will rise, fall, or split into developing product lines. You even know of desperately needed products not even invented—products you know promise unbelievable sales potential once they hit the market. This insight is precious. Corporate giants like General Motors and General Mills don't even draw sales leads that are this accurate and effective. They pay enormous amounts for such factual information and still run the risk of dry leads.

With your eardrum literally resting on the soundwave of consumer needs, decisions about what topic to propose or products to sell should be relatively easy. The toughest decision is not *what to sell, as much as whether you have the willingness to sell it.* Reluctance for any reason to pursue your marketing plan can sabotage you. It stops the flow of creative juices and puts off until tomorrow—or even later—a fabulous idea dying for action. A way around the procrastination trap is defusing, once and for all, the myths of self-marketing.

MYTHS OF SELF-MARKETING

Myth 1: Product Promotion Is Expensive

"Cost efficiency" is the buzzword of the 1990s and implies minimizing expenses while maximizing your output. You are already judiciously managing your budget, prioritizing expenses and letting the remainder be spent on self-indulging activities, personal recreation, clothes, and family holidays. Where does a budget for product promotion fit into all of this?

Intuitively, you think it doesn't. You don't want to exceed your office budget and would hate to dip into the family savings. The feeling is that costs for book proposals and undertaking the campaign of calling publishers and producers is entirely too expensive. Forget it. Fears of overspending on tight budgets and still failing seem imprudent.

Truth

Projected expenditures for proposal setup and publisher shopping are greatly inflated. Costs to actually write your proposal and expeditiously contact prospective buyers via facsimile and e-mail are minuscule. We're talking here about a phone bill of less than $50.00 and proposal preparation done for free. Unless you need a script doctor editing your document, expect your in-house labor costs to be pennies. In comparing your unpaid time writing a proposal to your paid time seeing patients, you may lose money, but regarding the proposal and letter writing time as part of your time allotted to clerical paperwork, allows you to treat it in your schedule as noncompensation.

Myth 2: Product Promotion Is Time Consuming

You may fear that time spent on proposal writing and finding buyers will eat away precious hours from the clock. Time constraints already exist in keeping appointments punctual and regulating other tasks around the appointments. The idea of infusing a new project in tightly managed hours seems preposterous.

Truth

Much of the homework needed for a solid, persuasive proposal already is in your head. You've compiled it over years of treatment delivery and have it down to a science. Converting that introspective database into a document, accompanied by a standard inquiry letter occupies less time than mowing the lawn. True, on outdoor chores, the beginning and end points are more readily visible. On constructing proposals, length from outset to finish is vague if you're not sure what to write, how long to make it, and whether the content is compelling. With a blueprint for writing followed carefully and few exceptions made, you can predict, control, and be happy with your time allotments. Even direct phone calls to publishers and producers can follow a prewritten script rather than be extemporaneous. This saves oodles of time.

Myth 3: Product Promotion Is Risky

Are you a gambler? No? Then, in your conservative mindset it seems outrageously irrational to plot a course for doomsday. The entire project from start to finish seems awfully risky in three ways. First, you immediately assume the market is saturated with self-help and recovery books and that a new one cannot possibly make a difference. Recycled versions of current bestsellers is not your idea of original writing. Second, you presume there is no publisher alive who will consider an unpublished author let alone an unknown professional. Although educated with a master's, doctorate, or medical degree, you conclude these credentials are a dime a dozen, outdone by many household names such as Dr. Ruth and Dr. Joyce Brothers. Who are you in the face of these celebrities? Third, you anticipate with great trepidation the ultimate rejection letter reminding you that, as you knew it, your idea was a waste of time.

Truth

Nothing is a waste of time. A closer inspection of actual higher-degree recipients in mental health is most eye-opening—you're actually a minority. Advanced degrees are still statistically uncommon in this day of college-bound high school graduates. After a four-year stint, graduates gladly board the career ship headed for high-paying, dollar-seeking jobs, such as those in international exchange, banking, the stock market, and financial advisement. Few undergraduate psychology or health services majors are embarking on graduate studies either due to prohibitive costs or unwillingness to devote another three to six years earning a doctorate. Given this unflattering outlook, I would say your degree and career is not a dime a dozen but more of a rare commodity.

As for saturation levels, think again. Proliferation of how-to and self-improvement books is due to a market demand. People want these things. Reading, whether from the printed page or on computer, is at an all-time high and even teens are flocking to recovery shelves. Books with similar names on similar topics may at first seem redundant. But there is a reason for redundancy. Devoted buyers want titles that hit home with their emotional problems. Titles sounding entirely different from what buyers want, although covering the same topic, are left behind. This creates a semantic expedition for the right power words to capture audiences' attention without infringing on another author's copyright. Can it be done? You bet!

Take, for instance, books on success. There are hundreds of them. A nifty bestseller took the American public by surprise years ago, titled *The One Minute Manager.* Spinoffs from this hot-cooking title immediately were overnight sensations, even though they all stole the opening phrase, "The One-Minute . . . ." My book called *Sixty Seconds to Success* enjoyed its own success on the coattails of this bestseller's book title and hopefully so will my next book due out soon called *One-Minute Secrets to Feeling Great.*

But is there anything new in these books not said before? That's a good question. A cursory reading of each "success" book that enjoys moderate sales will reveal an unusual conclusion. They are really different. Words and ideas actually are dissimilar. This is because the authors did their homework. First, they were alert to competitive books and only secured a publication because they showed how their books *must be different.*

Second, authors are the Christopher Columbuses of today's new frontier. They all want to discover a new world and lead an annual pilgrimage to this center of Mecca. To do this, they must have original material inscribed by their own peculiar theoretical ideas. (See Fried, 1994; and Fried and Schultis, 1995.) This will be true no matter what the pop-psychology book is that you read.

Myth 4: Product Promotion Is Complex

Sorting through the paradox of proposal writing, publisher contacts, negotiations, and other peripheral planning stages seems so complex. Who do you contact? What happens if they say yes? Consider the possibility of multiple, simultaneous submissions all receiving an affirmative "Okay, let's go ahead with publication." Now what? Which do you choose? Why? Disturbing questions such as these plague inexperienced writers who flirt with the idea of proposals but chicken out at the last moment. They get cold feet and figure, "It's too much to handle right now in my life."

Truth

Ever apply for a license? No, not your driver's license, but rather the state licensure for practicing your mental health specialty. Psychologists, social workers, rehabilitation counselors, nursing practitioners, psychiatrists–all of these professionals early in their careers muddled through the bureaucratic paper stack of application forms to obtain a license. Instructions on those forms are horrible. Judging from my state, your only chance is to contact a clerk in the state office and hope he or she will clarify the mess. If the clerk can't help, it means rereading the perplexed instructions until somehow and in some way you can make heads or tails of it. Now, that's what I call complex; I'm sure you would agree.

But complexity or not, you prevailed. You fought the intrusively stupid instructions, tolerated the moronic replies clerks gave on the telephone ("I'm sorry, I can't help you, I'm just answering the phone for this person."). You even persisted like a trooper until every single, solitary "I" was dotted and "T" was crossed. Never did it cross your mind while scuba diving in muddy waters that you should go up for air and not come back down. You never gave up. And why? You couldn't give up. Winning was the only outcome. Securing that license meant you could begin professionally after years of education.

The strange irony is that license application challenges and proposal and manuscript writing are truly two peas in the same pod. Once you feel inspired with ideas for a book, magazine article, software, or TV or business video, passion takes over with zeal.

You persevere over towering obstacles because *you simply want to achieve your goal that badly.* Partly due to deep commitment, and partly because you honestly believe you're a talented enough writer, you plunge forth feet first realizing the confusions of *what to do* will disappear once you actually begin doing, just as it did during the licensing ordeal.

Myth 5: Product Promotion Is for Publicists, Not Me

Avid readers of "empowerment" books pick up an idea very quickly: competency comes from delegating duties to people. Farm out assignments, tasks, and anything threatening to completely consume your limited planning time. In that spirit, providers may view proposal writing and product marketing as tasks better left to experts who do these activities for a living. Just as, they assume, computer repairs are deferred to a serviceperson, so too should book, magazine, and software writing be deferred to a publicist or packaging company that is already wearing the right shoes to walk the bumpy terrain.

Truth

There is wisdom, no doubt, in allocating unwanted tasks to people who thrive on the task's complications. I, for one, fully respect this practice. In writing proposals and publisher contacts, however, using the middle-man approach backfires. Except for rare occasions (as will be seen below), intermediaries are useless during initial stages of proposal and contract development since they cannot fully express the energy and acumen you bring to a topic. Publishers and producers want a firsthand pitch from the horse's mouth. They want it from you. That way, they can read or hear your genuine emotions as predictive of a book's impact on the buying public. Emotions that are translated by the salesmanship tongue of agents and publicists lose the vital force underlying the book's origins and sculpted form. Publishers in effect want to hear a catharsis; they acutely listen to the author's intimately personal reasons until the right chord is struck and a deal is made.

Myth 6: Product Promotion Is Frustrating and Leads to Failure

Earlier I alluded to patience. How patient are you? You know how tolerant you are at experimenting with new projects. A plumber you are not. A landscaper—you tried and definitely are not. A car mechanic—forget it, don't even try, not even to change the oil. Each attempt at doing a project yourself wound up being the worst nightmare of your life. Parts of the puzzle simply did not go together, even when you forcefully added glue to the pieces. If writing proposals or tinkering around with magazine, book, software, or video products promises to be anything like failures in the past, shut the door on the project right now.

Truth

There is a weird formula that I learned of the hard way for embarking on new projects. Believe me, I didn't stumble over this concept until mid-adulthood, after shouting obscenities at my mistakes for many years. It goes like this:

$$E + E = E. \ldots \text{ or } E^3$$

Error + Effort = Excellence

"E-cubed," you might say, represents a trajectory of learning stages that everybody must go through. Sorry, no cheating is allowed. There simply is no way around the fact that failure is inevitable when sticking your neck out in a new territory where you don't have an adequate roadmap.

My wife says she hates taking the travel agency's map on vacations because she prefers "winging it." She uses her intuitive mental compass. Well, that's her talent, not mine. My mental compass is out of order and I wouldn't trust it. Even if I did, I may still flounder around in circles. The same is absolutely true with writing and marketing your manuscripts. Failure is *not the catastrophic price you pay for trying. It is the normal obstacle you confront in learning a new skill—a skill that eventually produces winning results.*

As with any life challenge, *errors and effort* are the brothers Gemini whose impetus gets you over the hump of hating yourself.

Rather than be a perfectionist, forget about an editor's rejection and let your creative abilities surface for a change. At worst, you'll mutter to yourself, "I told you so, I knew you wouldn't get published." At best, you'll be surprised how exceptionally gifted you are at constructing highly marketable materials.

WHY YOU CAN MARKET YOURSELF

Putting myths of promotion aside, you may feel eagerly motivated to really give writing proposals and product marketing a try. Why not? Now is your chance. With a wealth of experience under your belt, you can contribute highly perceptive ideas individually wrapped to meet a particular reading audience. That's what tips off the publisher or producer that you are the "Real McCoy." Just how do you "wrap" proposal and products for this effect? In four ways.

Four important ingredients go into the recipe for outstanding proposals. They act as the backbone holding together the proposal and effectively pushing it ahead of other proposals in the deep pile on the editor's desk. You'll achieve an editor's review if the proposal contains (1) language of persuasion, (2) empirical support for the product, (3) credentials for publicity, and (4) efficiency on deadlines.

Language of Persuasion

Language of persuasion refers to the masterful art of speaking in editors' English. Journalists in touch with editorial styles and accustomed to tabloid writing have an intuitive feel for this. Scholars don't. Editors' English is where the sentences and paragraphs are short and the vocabulary is easy to understand. Polemical phrases and words frequently appropriate a lecture, for example, are inappropriate for editors. While intellectually elevated language is compelling proof of writer integrity for academic publishers, in the nonfiction trade this eloquence is annoying.

Drop the $25,000 words when describing a concept, for example, in explaining "guilt." A scholarly way is to argue that "unhealthy defense mechanisms interfere with self-expression resulting in a decomposition of the person's self-esteem." Now, as experienced clinicians, reading that last phrase may seem like common sense. Even in conversation with another colleague, this explanation may flow smoothly between speaker and listener without any communication gap.

But now try laying this heavy explanation on your patients. Try, even, patients with an eighth grade or less education who are prime sufferers of guilt and who you'd expect would grasp your meaning. Well, guess again. They may smile politely, but understanding you is another story. They probably don't have a clue to what your saying.

Here's how you would translate the phrase into editors' English: *When people get defensive, it later bothers them so much they may get depressed.* Semantically simpler words replace jargon and the sentence flows easier. Though, many complain, simplification may lose the meaning of a word and may even obscure the concepts further, that is only true if you want readers to have a technical understanding—this *is the purpose of academic writing.*

In trade writing, however, readers want fast and simple solutions spared of "why it works" and without the scientific or operational language defining the ideas. They want the *Reader's Digest* version"–a down-to-earth, straightforward message on how to be a better person.

Proposals scribed in this matter-of-fact language alert the editor to your audience sensitivity and ability to write clearly, understandably, and for mass consumption. What makes this writing style persuasive is that it jumps out on the page in bright, shiny colors in contrast to heavy, dark scholarly blotches (see Chapter 4 for more on writing style).

Empirical Support for the Product

In oral dissertation defenses and paper presentations at conferences, collegial input is rough. Your peers are painfully skeptical of your *empirical data supporting your research.* Questions are asked about sample selection, methods of assessment, evaluation instruments, data analysis, and other details of the study.

Well, here's the good news. That is not what editors and producers want. They could care less if in deriving results you used a chi-square or T-test or whether you applied a time series or single case research design. What they *do care about it* is whether your facts and theories have overall empirical validity. They will trust your innate wisdom and assume you used tools of the trade in producing your ideas. They rightfully or wrongly assume that, were they to be called on the carpet by media vultures, you'd be ready to bail them out.

On one book, for example, where I recently acted as ghostwriter and co-author, facts pertained to previously classified government documents obtained through Freedom of Information (FOI) requests. Confidential documents surprisingly revealed incredibly incriminating information about our government's activity during wartime. It reopened a can of worms most of the public believed was shut tight and buried (Naujoks and Ruben, in press). While the publisher trusted our data collection and even interpretation of these documents, he took the legal precaution of having us put our "ducks in order" just in case government troublemakers or radical social groups rallied at his doorstep. That meant that we had to systematically categorize our data in such a way that, if necessary, an audit would show we did our homework.

But, honestly, does this happen all the time? No. This is the rare exception to the rule for most nonfiction trade writing. In most cases, publishers and producers simply want the reassurance that expressed viewpoints have some empirical foundation, whatever it is and however you obtained it.

Credentials for Publicity

A question frequently asked in proposal writing is this: Will my academic degrees make a difference? The answer is yes, big time. Credibility is the heartbeat of believability. When Doctor So and So says on national TV that seasonal depression infects 40 to 50 percent of men and women living in gloomy climates, believe me: that advice becomes gospel. People move to Florida.

Degrees speak with authority. A book authored by Dr. Somebody will carry more prestige than a book by a nondoctor, unless that nondoctor author has a public image. Such authors have a track record in some specialty commanding a large sympathetic audience. Consider prime-time recovery books. Readers of books on adult children of alcoholics, domestic assault, and codependency care less about author credentials than they do about the material. Ideas must accurately pinpoint their inner hurt. Authors at bachelor's and master's levels whose words prick a thick artery of emotion in their readers can enjoy publishing success equal to that of their higher-degreed colleagues.

Publishers and producers still make a stink about credentials for one reason: *to sell books.* They actually would not quibble over bachelor's- or master's-degreed professionals having as much if not more knowledge than a doctorate professional, but they know the difficulty in public relations. Selling to an impulse-purchasing public means selling a quick fix. Respected authors draw their readers in. Less known or first-time authors without higher advanced degrees run amuck. They may need to initially write a book for less discriminating audiences and then use their book as leverage.

Clarify for the publisher or producer exactly what your credentials are for publishing, how much you've presented at conferences, and what you do in public. Be objective and accurate, but don't be shy. Humbling yourself will only disqualify your true community impact and underestimate your potential to reach wider audiences. Explain, for example, that you're a regular presenter at several county PTO or school board meetings, that you are a fixture in training leadership at religious and secular weekend retreats, or that you've consulted to extensive parenting groups on Attention Deficit Hyperactivity Disorder (ADHD), Sudden Infant Death Syndrome (SIDS), or other recovery groups. Extent of community activity, including public exposure on TV, radio, or news media, is a definite plus in building your credibility record.

Efficiency on Deadlines

The age of electronic publishing is upon us. Today, publishers with sophisticated computer technology move a manuscript faster in production than ever before. Diskette submissions with manuscript already typeset and in format saves months of typesetting and copyediting. Diskettes sent as file attachments over the internet rapidly transmit documents directly into computers, and editors do not have to fool around with software conversions. In all, production time is expeditious when author and publisher coordinate their manuscript-linking technologies and meet mutually set deadline dates.

That is why you want your proposal to explicitly comment on your computer capacities and your personal history of meeting deadlines. Naturally, as busy clinicians, report-writing deadlines are a weekly occurrence. Providers who procrastinate drafting reports not only disrupt a "process" (for example, meetings at schools, child custody determination in court, diagnosed disability for social security), but in the long run, also lose an important referral base. A fast turnaround time between assignment and deadline is preferred. It is also the sign of the type of author that publishers and producers are looking for. Speed and accuracy of delivering a product on time or even before deadline *proves to the publisher that you are reliable, market-conscious, and highly motivated.*

Sad to say, some publishers and producers of mass market products still use antiquated systems of production. Older equipment and hard-copy editing delay release of your prized possession. That can be very frustrating for "Johnny-on-the-spot" professionals who are almost obsessive about deadlines and fulfilling their part of the contract—and then some. Annoying as it is, be patient. Longer production by no means undervalues the editor's respect for you or your book.

REFERENCES

Braus, P. (1992). Selling self-help (marketing self-help programs). *American Demographics, 14,* 48.

Fried, S.B. (1994). *American popular psychology: An interdisciplinary research guide.* New York: Garland Press.

Fried, S.B. and Schultis, G.A. (1995). *The best self-help and self-awareness books: A topic-by-topic guide to quality information.* Chicago, IL: American Library Association.

Naujoks, A. and Ruben, D.H. (in press). *Hitler's revenge.* Salt Lake City, UT: Northwest Publishing.

Starker, S. (1990). Self-help books: Ubiquitous agents of health care. *Medical Psychotherapy, 3,* 187-194.

Chapter 3

Rapid Ways to Reach Your Market

BOOK PROPOSALS

Proposal writing is a headache if you make one mistake: the mistake in thinking that publishers will only consider your idea if the submission includes a sample chapter. Economy of time prevents publishers from delving into each submission and reading 50 to 100 double-spaced, typed manuscript pages. Instead, reviews are cursory. Cover pages, along with a five to six-page proposal are flipped through and attached chapters are put aside. By examining the proposal, publishers instantly know if authors *have writing talents for lay readership.*

In Chapter 9 of *Publicity for Mental Health Clinicians* (Ruben, 1995, pp. 138-145), detailed descriptions are given of the proposal from cover letter to contents. Here, I wish to supplement that information with updated facts and tips relative to market changes in the last year.

Cover Letter

Once upon a time, hot-breaking news stories caused publishers to hold their breath. Stories had to be big and had to be important. Discovery of the decomposed body of celebrity model Margaux Hemingway or resignation of controversial Bosnian-Serb leader Radovan Karadzic were good examples. Those would stop the presses. E-mail pitches from biographers would promise a two-week turnaround time from contract to a finished book. That quick? Yes. And dollar signs flashed in front of publishers' eyes.

The faster publishers produced and distributed high-profile books to booksellers, the faster their profits grew. However, eagerness to capitalize on fast cash-earning biography books took a temporary nosedive when the media snubbed the book industry. Lately, for instance, ex-FBI agent Gary Aldrich's new book *Unlimited Access* bled to death in low ratings when national TV shows canceled this rebel's interview appearance.

And why? Timing of his book release was too close to the 1996 presidential campaign. It smeared both Democratic and Republican candidates, burning both ends of the candle and making author Aldrich appear the only hero. Well, it didn't work.

But is controversy really bad? No. Aldrich's book is bound to stimulate curiosity in news-seeking readers wondering what the fuss is all about. Still, it called into question the ethics of publishing and the author's credibility.

That is why fast assignments of books, even on nationally hot issues, is on the downside. Publishers want to marinate over book proposals to project a strong marketing plan. If they can picture one in their mind, they will send you a contract.

That accounts for two new variations of the cover letter. The first is called the "trust-me" letter (see Figure 3.1). Trust-me letters consist of four main paragraphs and have an opening line that powerfully highlights a strong feature about the author. If you've published before, say it. If you're a renowned workshop leader, say it. Next is a paragraph assuring the publisher that this expertise will guarantee follow-through and pay off in the short run. The second paragraph briefly pitches the book, focusing on its purpose and audience angle. The third paragraph reminds the publisher of what you said at the outset. It reiterates your credentials not only in writing style but also in terms of marketing the book. Last, be sure to indicate enclosures you have sent along.

Figure 3.1 has one other unusual entry. It is from a publicist working in my office who, at the time, handled correspondence. One advantage of this is having another person glamorize your capability without you sounding arrogant. However, toned down a bit, letter and signature can be from the author.

A second variation attempts to get two ideas for the price of one letter. It's called the "implosive approach" (see Figure 3.2). Here, consider presenting several ideas simultaneously in a letter. By analogy, think of a mutual market fund. Decline of one stock is

FIGURE 3.1. Letter to publisher with specific book proposal

BEST IMPRESSIONS INTERNATIONAL INCORPORATED

4211 OKEMOS ROAD, SUITE 22, OKEMOS, MICHIGAN 48864, U.S.A.
PHONE or FAX: 517-347-0944; PHONE: 1-800-595-BEST

March 13, 1995

Ms. Lynn Brown, Publisher
Zebra & Pinnacle Books
850 Third Avenue
New York, NY 10022

Dear Ms. Brown:

Finally, a seasoned author whose book you can count on!

Wouldn't it be nice if your author already published several self-help books, had established media contacts, and knew the ropes of book production? That's why Dr. Doug Ruben's latest book will probably be the safest investment you ever made.

We invite you to consider Dr. Ruben's latest book, *Smart Sex: Choosing Who, When, Where, and How Much* for publication. This is a practical survival kit on how to meet, date, and romance sexual partners. Chapters spell out secrets on finding eager partners, why they are eager, and what turns partners off. Plus, common dating mistakes that sabotage sex are identified, as well as powerful solutions that stimulate sexual drives. Guidelines offer rapid ways to arouse trust, emotional love, and focus on *who, when, and where, and how much to make love.*

And all with Dr. Ruben's unique "you-can-do-it-too" style. Recently on *Donahue!,* Dr. Ruben's flair for self-helpers won him national acclaim for *No More Guilt: Ten Steps to a Shame-Free Life, Bratbusters: Say Goodbye to Tantrums and Disobedience,* and *Avoidance Syndrome: Doing Things Out of Fear.* After 30-plus books, Dr. Ruben's media network ranges from doing talk-show circuits to producing TV shows.

Knowing his superb track record, it pays to consider *Smart Sex* for publication. Enclosed for your initial review is a prospectus. Please call, fax, or write to request a sample chapter. We look forward to your reply.

Thank you for your time.

Sincerely,

Paul Smith, Publicist
Best Impressions International Inc.

FIGURE 3.2. Letter to publisher with various book proposal ideas

BEST IMPRESSIONS INTERNATIONAL INCORPORATED

4211 OKEMOS ROAD, SUITE 22, OKEMOS, MICHIGAN 48864, U.S.A.
FAX or PHONE: 517-347-0944; PHONE: 1-800-595-BEST; local 347-1811
E-MAIL: mjruben@aol.com

February 7, 1996

Editor
Aanvil Press
P.O. Box 881
Booth Bay Harbor, ME 04538

Dear Acquisitions Editor:

Our literary and teleproductions agency represents screenwriters/authors with theme fiction and nonfiction (historical, biographical, self-help) texts. .

Currently we have properties available for your editorial review. Titles and loglines are presented below. We'd be happy to e-mail or fax one-page summaries of each property. Let us know if you would like sample chapters from any of these titles. We also would be happy to receive your newsletter/catalogs updating us on your editorial needs.

Thanks –   Doug Ruben, President
             Best Impressions International Inc.
             4211 Okemos Road, Suite 22
             Okemos, MI 48864

Properties for your editorial review:

Wanna Get Even? (nonfiction): Brief youth survival pamphlet/workbook against violence, teaching basic ways to respond under threats of fear and intimidation, and helping parents understand what kids go through. (requires an advance)

Smart Sex: Choosing Who, When, Where, and How Much (nonfiction): Handbook for X-generation singles and divorcees looking for male selection without repeating relationship failures on merry-go-round of highs and lows. Explicit how-to steps guide readers through methods on being a "choosy shopper" in the sexual marketplace. (requires an advance)

Little Miss Breadwinner: And the Crumbs She Dates (nonfiction): Power advice from Playboy model and actress Martha Smith (and associates) on how to stop the vicious cycle of uncaring lovers sponging off your emotions. Provides practical stepwise skills to avoid down-dating traps and enjoy healthy partners. (requires an advance)

Blood Rights (horror): Based on a recent news story of a man abducting young girls and keeping them in his basement mausoleum; filled with satanic and high-suspense thrills.

Nellie's Law (fiction, western): La Femme western of gunslinging heroine taken to the high road in revenge of her slain kin. Sort of Dirty Harry, female style.

A Toothy Tale (children's illustrated book): Beautiful story of Tyrone the gentle dinosaur, who is miserably upset over other dinosaurs' rejection of him whenever he opens his mouth. His teeth were not right, but steps he takes to overcome social rejection and build friendships are inspiring and delightfully contagious for young readers.

The Female Trap (fiction, suspense): Romantic deception draws in unsuspecting bystander until he realizes he's become obsessively attracted to a woman, devouring his time, life, and goals. In the end, she reveals her secret of baiting him, but he's already bitten by the passion bug.

Triumph (fiction, romance): Riveting Romeo and Juliet romance between Mexican football hero and Anglo-Saxon female from wealthy family caught in triangle of racial prejudice, loyalty, and endless love. Against dismal odds, the relentless couple's marriage blasts through family tensions, finally winning respect.

Silent Cries (fiction, suspense): Murder-mystery romance revolves around brutal rape, murder, and a detective obsessed with finding suspects. The book chronicles victim's life as suspense builds through investigation and courtroom scenes. Story wraps around pulsating intrigue, sex, violence, and visions of justice.

The Franchese Covenant (fiction, historical): Traces origins of two mafia families and decades of sordid rivalry. Two families fighting for power undermined by a talking killer gives energy to the plot and keeps the reader glued to the book. Scheme follows the families through their business manipulations and eventual uniting of forces.

Wounds of Hate (contemporary fiction): Gangland in San Jose follows a crime-fighting teacher determined to beat the skinheads in their violent town.

Jenny Dog and Son of Light (fiction, wilderness): Imagine "rescue Lassie" in this mountain adventure of canine love as emergency teams find lost survivors in the wilderness.

Tale Teller: Great Short Stories from Masterworks of Literature (nonfiction, supplemental reader for secondary, college): Top anthology of worldwide, famous authors from Dickens to Dostoyevsky, but in condensed, short stories able to be read within eight minutes per story. Appeals to Generation X, low attention span students who can now absorb classic literature within minutes. Stories cover human interest, psychological tales, religious tales, historical tales, allegorical tales, tales in poetry, classical tales, medieval tales, humorous tales, fantasy tales, and tales of horror.

offset by other rising stocks, resulting in an overall gain. Here, the rising stocks are other fiction or nonfiction trade options proposed to a publisher without sending any attachments such as a proposal. The letter stands alone, introducing each book using a "logline." A logline is a brief, one to four-sentence description of the book. Frequently, you'll find loglines used in television guides explaining a movie or TV show. Loglines are succinct devices to induce publisher interest in seeing a proposal or sample chapters.

Proposal

Proposals are the authoritative roadmap to pages of your book. A proposal is a four to five-page document broken down into five parts. The first part is the *general description and specification*. Second is the *length of manuscript and estimated completion date*. Third is the *table of contents*. Fourth is *competitive market*. And fifth is *about the author*. Again, barring repetition from my previous book in this series, I have only highlighted key changes you may wish to make on a typical proposal, as shown in Figure 3.3.

General Description and Specification

This brief narrative overviews the content and compelling role the book serves in the self-help industry. Who will it help? How? Explain the chapters generically, pointing out exceptional qualities of high market potential. In addition, be sure the opening paragraph clearly covers the following:

1. *What area of human need does it tap?*
2. *What makes this book so irresistible?*
3. *What major feature separates this book from competitors' books?*

Area of human need entails how this book taps right into the five pulses of buyer-mentality. These include *vanity, greed, power, success,* and *love*. True, you can expand these to include all seven deadly sins and even broaden the list further with sublists detailing how people indulge in each of these vices. Still, no matter how you turn or twist them around, dictating consumer shopping instincts are these basic human needs.

FIGURE 3.3. Complete proposal to be sent to book publisher

PROSPECTUS

Smart SEX!
Choosing Who, When, Where, and How Much

Douglas H. Ruben, PhD
Best Impressions International Inc.
Okemos, Michigan

Contents

1. **General Description and Specification**

2. **Length of Manuscript and Estimated Completion Date**

3. **Table of Contents**

4. **Competitive Market**

5. **About the Author**

FIGURE 3.3 (continued)

(2) *Smart SEX! Choosing Who, When, Where, and How Much*

1. *General Description and Specification*

Smart SEX! Choosing Who, When, Where, and How Much proposes the first complete survival kit on how to meet, date, and romance sexual partners. Chapters spell out secrets on finding eager partners, why they are eager, and what turns partners off. Common dating mistakes that sabotage sex are identified, followed by concrete solutions to avoid these mistakes and stimulate sexual drives. Steps to enhance affection take a different twist: readers get verbal and nonverbal guidelines that instantly arouse trust, emotional love, and sexual dependency. Less focus is concentrated on *how* to make love, and more focus on *who, when, where,* and *how much* to make love: this maximizes sexual opportunities. Rapidly effective techniques take the mystery out of mate searching. Strategies open doors of opportunity for dating singles, for couples in sexual distress, and for individuals tired of repeating bad relationships. Now they'll have at their fingertips a blueprint for dependable love connections.

2. *Length of Manuscript and Estimated Completion Date*

Manuscript length estimated at 250 to 300 double-spaced pages (excluding front matter, back matter). Estimated completion date is six months to one year following contractual agreement. Considering computer capacities on the Macintosh/IBM and laser printer, photo-ready preparation is available based on higher advances against royalty sales and higher royalty percentage on net sales. On computer, manuscript can be completed in Microsoft Word (5.0) or Pagemaker.

3. *Table of Contents*

From the Author

Chapter 1: Who wants sex?

     a. How to spot sexually eager types
     b. Why smarter doesn't equal sexier
     c. Why more attractive doesn't equal sexier
     d. Why more "experienced" doesn't equal sexier
     e. Drawbacks of sexually eager types
     f. Why eager types make you less eager

(3) *Smart SEX! Choosing Who, When, Where, and How Much*

Chapter 2: When is the "right time" for sex?

    a. Why in the morning?
    b. Why in the middle of the day, or during work or school?
    c. Why at night?
    d. Prime situations for sex
    e. Lousy situations for sex

Chapter 3: Why does "No, leave me alone!" drive you crazy?

    a. No relief
    b. No dignity
    c. No trust
    d. No love
    e. No romance
    f. No friendship
    g. Feel ugly
    h. Feel taken for granted
    i. Feel it's different from dating

Chapter 4: Why does your partner say "NO" to sex?

    a. Bad habits
    b. Bad timing
    c. Bad experiences
    d. No experiences
    e. Bad method
    f. Fears and modesty
    g. Pain
    h. Anger
    i. It's better alone
    j. Somebody else
    k. Waste of time
    l. Tired
    m. Too much too soon
    n. Inconvenient contraception

Chapter 5: What not to do when sex is refused

    a. Take it personally
    b. Fake it
    c. Surrender to defeat
    d. Fantasize about sex with somebody else
    e. Have sex with somebody else
    f. Peep at somebody else
    g. Threaten separation or divorce
    h. Masturbate

FIGURE 3.3 (continued)

(4) *Smart SEX! Choosing Who, When, Where, and How Much*

i. New pornography
j. Fantasize about rape

Chapter 6: What to do when sex is refused

More Talking
a. What to talk about
b. How to talk about it
c. Ways to defuse arguments
d. Ways to comfort fears
e. Ways to reinforce effort

More Affection
a. Start where it's at
b. Okay "touch" areas
c. Touch in front of kids, other family
d. Rules about when touch is annoying

More Risks
a. Inventory of "can't do's"
b. Minor experiments with touch
c. Share control
d. How to relax
e. Small steps to excitement

More Convenience
a. Different times for sex
b. Different contraception
c. Different ways to approach sex

Chapter 7: Where is it OKAY to have sex?

a. Safe places
b. Risky places
c. Why risky places get addictive
d. Why risky places lose excitement
e. How to be creative

Chapter 8: How much sex is too much sex?

a. Are you a one-a-day vitamin?
b. Are you a frequent flyer?
c. Can you go without sex for an hour?
d. When does erotic turn neurotic?
e. Power-up for playtime

(5) Smart SEX! Choosing Who, When, Where, and How Much

4. Competitive Market (the "angle")

The good news is that few sex books on this specific topic are on the market. Few exist because the topic is very specialized and requires a firm understanding of behavioral principles, sexual hang-ups, and marital therapy. Most authors get one or the other idea correct, but overall methods are incomplete. *Smart SEX!* deliberately combines all three issues. David Rubin's *Everything You Always Wanted to Know About Sex, Any Woman Can!* and *How to Get More Out of Sex* stirred controversy over two decades ago, opening doors for Stanton Peele's highly compelling *Sex and Addiction*. But that was almost eight years ago. Since then, sex-recovery books have stolen a chunk of the reader's market, with books like *Hope and Recovery: 12-Step Guide for Healing from Compulsive Sexual Behavior* (1987) and *LoveMaps* (1986). No other serious competitor focuses on sexual behavior-change approaches for couples. Most of these recovery manuals also overlook why substitutes for healthy marital intimacy *don't work–and why. Smart SEX!* dives headfirst into these reasons with remedies for every person to apply.

5. About the Author

Dr. Douglas Ruben is an addictions and family therapist and national consultant in media psychology. His seminars on recovery and how to "rate your date" cover the entire Midwest, and he has appeared in two national infomercials (one produced by Guthy-Renker). Dr. Ruben is author and co-author of over 30 books and over 100 professional articles. Among his recent books are *No More Guilt: 10 Steps to a Shame-Free Life*; *Bratbusters: Say Goodbye to Tantrums and Disobedience*; *Avoidance Syndrome*; *Doing Things Out of Fear*; *Family Recovery Companion*; *60 Seconds to Success*; and *One Minute Secrets to Feeling Great*. He wrote the blueprint for other authors with *Your Public Image: TV, Radio and Print Media in Clinical Practice* (due out in Fall). Recently on *Donahue!*, Dr. Ruben frequently appears on TV and radio talk shows from coast to coast, including *Kelly & Co* (Detroit), *Good Company* (Minneapolis), *Morning Exchange* (Cleveland), *AM Northwest* (Portland, OR), *Conversation with Ed Clancy* (New Orleans), and *Top of the Morning* (Birmingham, AL). He is also the associate producer of *The Celebrity Golf Show*, airing on TCI channels. Full vita available upon request.

The book *Smart Sex* clearly falls into the category of *love*. Notice, too, this book bypasses the orthodoxy of how-to instructions on lovemaking and is proposing a taboo look at *who, when, where, and how much* to make love. That doesn't feel right for some people, but it isn't those people that I'm trying to sell the book to. For Middle America, finding a sexual (not dating) partner verges on heresy.

That's why publishers may love the idea; it teases the public. Buyers are tempted by lustful fantasies to taste the forbidden fruit: the book. Two years ago, Madonna's book *Sex*, which among other things details sexually explicit lovemaking positions, took the market by storm. Despite brutal controversy and moral upheaval, the book scored big at cash registers.

Length of Manuscript and Estimated Completion Date

Little has changed in this category except for page length and computer facility. Self-help and recovery books are shorter, more how-to than expository. Double-spaced page lengths vary from 250 to 300 pages for a produced 100- to 150-page book. Most trade publishers can convert your software into their software and can change fonts and point size according to their specifications. A new standard is to transmit part or all of your manuscript through 14.4- or 28.8-speed modems or through e-mail in a text (".txt") file that publishers can download directly into their programs. Meeting this high-tech challenge may or may not earn you bonus points in your contract, but it will certainly speed up production time and build a mutually helping publisher-author relationship.

Table of Contents

As usual, list the major heading and subheadings of chapter content. All headings should have a "byte" or imaginative use of words or phrases enticing readers in seconds. Note the subheadings under Chapter 1: Who wants sex? of "a. How to spot sexually eager types," or "f. Why eager types make you less eager." I will guarantee that barflies and dating-scene regulars looking around for how to decode sexual cues will immediately flip to those pages. Both topics appeal to their craving for power, lust, control, and physical dominance.

Competitive Market

Here is your soapbox. Pitch your angle on what your book offers that its competitors don't. A discussion about the shortcomings of current books in contrast to your bold improvements helps the publisher get a fix on whether your book can survive the market. Be confident, even a bit risky in criticizing similar books, in spite of their shelf life or whether you actually see good things in the book. Of course, every book has good things. That's why it was published. But you've hooked the publisher to read this far into your proposal and now you must pour on the sauce with as much self-boasting proof of your book as possible. Keep your reasons relevant to what your book has that others don't, and your electrifying words will not sound arrogant.

About the Author

Sell yourself. Now that the publisher or editor knows your book and has a mental picture of market direction, seal the deal with impeccable credentials. For seasoned authors or individuals who have a reputation, that is not hard to do. But what about newcomers? Are they out of luck? Do they fake it? How do they guarantee the editor will sign on the dotted line?

Here's how: by embellishing the one quality all newcomers already have in their practitioner capacity, that is, being effective therapists. You have no doubt developed specialties or a referral base around a highly skilled area in which you are recognized. If it's marriage therapy—fine. Talk about what you can do in marriage therapy that nobody this side of the equator can do. Say, for example, "Saved 35 divorce-pending couples in six months!" If it's pediatrics, toot your own horn with what you and your referrals keep telling you: "Turned bratty monsters into lovable kids in seven months." These "sound bytes" are magnets that draw editor attention and can earn you approval in no time. Turn the credibility of your clinical success into a billboard of words that testify to your genius and insight. It will work, believe me.

What's the Best Form of Communication?

Numerous channels of communication exist to reach editors and publishers. Rapidly transmittable media include facsimiles, e-mail, and phone calls. While regular mail (called "snail mail") is always at your disposal, trends away from conventional postal systems are rising in this evolving age of computers and electronic mail. Table 3.1 illustrates important advantages and disadvantages of using different modes of communication for book proposal submissions.

Two of the most functionally effective ways of communication are by facsimile and e-mail. Letters sent by facsimile reach the acquisitions editor immediately or are routed to *somebody in the editorial office* faster than by regular mail service. Faxes still

TABLE 3.1. Advantages and Disadvantages of Communication Media for Book Proposals

Type of Media	Advantages	Disadvantages
Snail mail	More detail given.	Slower reply time. Tendency to be verbose. Easier to lose in shuffle.
Fax	Strikes impulsive needs. Faster reply time. Cheaper than snail mail. Minimal effort for starters.	May be picked up later in day. Few or no details given. Less professional appearance.
E-mail	Fastest direct message. Retrievable day or night. Keeps focus on brevity.	No aesthetic quality. Delay in checking e-mail. Unable to send graphics.
Phone call	Get immediate answers. Establish contact person. More socially informal.	Nuisance to editors. Chance of poorly pitching good book. Refusal before book submitted.

prompt a sense of urgency in recipients who respond rapidly and succinctly. But brief replies provide direct answers of "yes" or "no" instead of perfunctory form letters and are scribed personally by the party you had in mind to reach. With e-mail, assuming editors log onto their server or read their e-mail, exchanges are usually warm, friendly, and done more leisurely.

Editors frequently read and reply to their e-mail after work at home and are less rushed by schedule pressures. E-mail also allows for an informal dialogue, not cluttered by letterhead stationary, graphics, or other "sweetening" elements hoping to sway interest.

MAGAZINE ARTICLE PROPOSALS

Magazine article proposals are another species entirely. Separate documents, such as the three- to five-page book proposal, are over-kill. Editors of busy tabloids are constantly on the lookout for uniquely innovative slants on topics endemic to their focus. For pets, training and breeding secrets are of special value. For the Boy Scouts, mature summer camping experiences told from a scout-leader perspective are desirable. In Christian parenting magazines, child management tips using insightful spiritual codes of conduct would be perfect. Each magazine strives for a new approach integrating known concepts or presenting concepts never heard before (Cool, 1986, 1987).

What editors want is a one-page inquiry clearly informing them of your topic, title, and why you are eminently qualified to write the paper (see Figure 3.4). Inquiry letters open with varying statements. You may draw upon a current news headline, tying it into your topic, or, compliments do just the trick. Praise for the magazine's fine quality of articles is always eye-catching. Laudatory remarks framed in the context of you, clinically, recommending these articles to patients especially indicates you are a loyal fan of the magazine.

In the second paragraph, state the subject of the article and which department or section of the magazine you wish it considered for. Magazines offer a variety of places for new freelancers. Smaller pieces of 300 to 500 words fit nicely in what they call "departments," which often include "sex and romance" or "family and

FIGURE 3.4. Cover letter to magazine publisher with proposal for article

March 4, 1996

Shannon V. McClintock, Editor
Atlanta Singles Magazine
Hudson Brooke Publishing Inc.
180 Allen Road, Suite 304N
Atlanta, GA 30328

Dear Shannon:

Enclosed please find a short manuscript on an exciting dating topic based on the books I've written. It's constructed in a format for rapid entertainment and consumption.

Please consider the manuscript for publication in *Atlanta Singles Magazine.*

Should you accept it, I'd be happy to forward a glossy black-and-white, 8 x 10 photograph of myself or additional author information.

Incidentally, I'd be happy to write a regular column/segments on RATE YOUR DATE, featuring hints, tips, and insider ways on securing healthy romances.

Let me know your thoughts. I can be reached at the address above or fax me at (517) 347-0944/347-1811, call at 1-800-595-BEST, or e-mail at mjruben @aol.com.

Looking forward to hearing from you.

Sincerely,

Douglas H. Ruben, PhD

marriage." Longer articles of 800 to 3,000 words qualify for a feature article. Editors are generally more selective about features and usually the product is assigned by an editor. Editors rarely accept unsolicited papers for features unless the topic is scalding hot or, serendipitiously, editors were actively soliciting this topic.

Finish the letter by politely inviting them to contact you by whatever mode of communication is faster.

What's the Best Form of Communication?

Reaching magazine editors is more difficult than reaching book editors and publishers. A hierarchical layer of editors usually construct the temple of tabloids, and keeping track of who is where is cumbersome. Phone-calls, even dialed directly to the editor's exchange, are futile. Nobody will answer it, or if they do, you'll get a revolving trip around the voice-mail mall. Table 3.2 discusses advantages and disadvantages of different modalities of contacting magazine decision makers.

Again, the winner is fax or e-mail. More editors rely on e-mail delivery than snail mail. For example, letters to the editor are increasingly sent by e-mail or through web-page bulletin boards. Retrieval is quicker, easier, produces less paper clutter, and response to e-mail senders is faster. While facsimiles are second best, delays may be excessive before the fax clerk routes incoming pages to their destinations. Lag time not only is frustrating but also builds false illusion that editors hate your idea and rejected it when, actually, they never read your letter.

SOFTWARE PROPOSALS

Inquiry letters are protocol in most submission packages. Software submissions are no exception. A cover letter briefly identifying who you are and briefly describing the attachment is plenty for starters. Spend more time on the proposal. Here, unlike book proposals, you are the owner of an idea only and possibly not the writer of the software program. As owner, you take the title of "developer." Software developers brainstorm new ideas and revise old

TABLE 3.2. Advantages and disadvantages of communication media for article proposals

Type of Media	Advantages	Disadvantages
Snail mail	Stationery shows credentials. More details for pitch.	Harder to pitch on paper. May get lost or rerouted. Delays ruin timely pieces. Too academic.
Fax	Piques interest quickly. Pitch can sound urgent. Faster editorial reply. Tap news story promptly.	May get rerouted or lost. May require telephone follow-up.
E-mail	More friendly. Pitch is succinct. Read day or night. Reach editor directly. Can verify when receiver read it.	Read once or twice weekly. Has unprofessional appearance.
Phone call	Rapport-building. Pitch is quick. Editorial reply is instant. Can start negotiating.	May not reach editor. Editor is impatient. Idea rejected coldly.

ideas for a snazzier, more dazzling interactive game, educational program, etc. Developers work in tandem with software programmers; these are the technicians competent in the logical language that runs a program. Some developers, themselves competent programmers, may provide the sequential mathematics necessary for running the software.

Most practitioners have neither the time nor inclination to learn complex programming language. I think my only "D" in college was in FORTRAN. I'm not sure my coursework in Basic fared much better. Still, remarkably easier programming tools are on the market for illiterates, many using icons (pictures) instead of long, complex word sequences or binary codes. These user-friendly programming alternatives greatly inspire neophytes but are still time-consuming and tax your patience. With time so scarce, I advise you stick with the software developing end.

Proposals run one to three pages and are divided into categories: *Identification, Brief summary, Basic steps, What developer can provide,* and *What developer needs from publisher* (see Figure 3.5). *Identification* is where your list your name, generic type of program (e.g., interactive, virtual reality, game), and projected style of computers on which the program would be playable (Macintosh, IBM, IBM-compatible). Reference can be more specific to Windows 3.0, Windows 95, DOS, Power Macintosh, or other operating systems.

Brief summary means just that. Here is a nutshell of the conceptual plot from beginning to end, in which you focus on unusual traps, tricks, or features likely to excite users of the program.

Basic steps lists the logical sequence of action by the player, which produces an orderly series of interactive effects. Technical specificity is not necessary here. Just keep it simple and storylike. Imagine, for example, giving directions to your office from the highway, naming all the key landmarks and cross streets. You would create a colorful mental roadmap for the listener who later has to implement this mental image in the car. Story-line steps are written with a similar image in mind; sketch out a blueprint visual that functions well enough for software publishers to mentally picture and determine if users (adults or children) will thoroughly enjoy it.

Two last sections include *What developers can provide* and *What developers need from publisher.* In the first case, enumerate on exactly what your expertise can lend to the project. Can you write the technical manual? the script of words used in the software? Can you prepare supplementary materials, for example, on history or process of litigation, which has educational value for users? In both proposals shown in Figure 3.5, instruction and game rules are not enough. As lawyer or therapist, game players need background details on how lawyers and therapists think, as well as tools of the trade. In one popular software game on performing medical surgery, for example, standard steps for surgery, basic medical school facts, and hints for diagnosis round out the background for informed readers to play more competitively.

FIGURE 3.5. Complete proposal to software company for software ideas

BEST IMPRESSIONS INTERNATIONAL INCORPORATED

4211 OKEMOS ROAD, SUITE 22, OKEMOS, MICHIGAN 48864, U.S.A.
PHONE/FAX: 517-347-0944; FAX: 517-349-1823; PHONE: 1-800-595-BEST;
E-MAIL: mjruben@aol.com

January 6, 1996

Mr. Don Laabs, Vice President
Product Development
The Software Toolworks
19808 Nordhoff Place
Chatsworth, CA 91311

Dear Mr. Laabs:

Thank you for requesting further information regarding the proposed software ideas of Final Verdict and My Therapist.

Enclosed for review, along with the evaluation agreement, are two initial program proposals.

Let us know your ideas on pursuing these games.

Very sincerely,

Douglas H. Ruben, PhD

Proposal #1

"Final Verdict"

Developers of Idea: Douglas H. Ruben, PhD and Marilyn J. Ruben
Type of Program: Interactive courtroom movie, in which you are the attorney
Computer Market: Macintosh, IBM, etc.

Brief Summary

"Final Verdict" brings real-life trial experience to the forefront of every person's imagination. This interactive software, much like Life & Death, places users in the role of trial attorney. Follow a series of choices and action-packed questions and answers from witnesses, the judge, and prosecution. Choose the level of difficulty: Beginner (e.g., traffic court, misdemeanor, etc.), Intermediate (felony cases, breaking and enterings, armed robbery), and Advanced (murder trials). Be the defense attorney and move from opening to closing argument to win your case. This may involve calling upon experts (medical, mental health, other categories) and examining and reexamining witnesses. Choose incriminating facts from the menu of evidence. Then, when it's the other attorney's turn to examine witnesses, get ready to press the mouse to signal objections to his line of questioning (menu of objections includes leading witness, badgering, etc.).

Be aware of the unsuspecting courtroom tricks. When litigating, keep an eye out for (a) the other attorney's objections and judge's decision (if overruled, you keep going; if sustained, you change line of inquiry); (b) the client's frantic outbursts (choose from menu of recovery, for example, remove client from courtroom, request court recess); and (c) funny things in the courtroom (crowd yells, somebody faints, etc.).

Basic Steps

Conceptually, this game proceeds in the following sequential order:

First, you attend "Law School" for briefing. Then, begin your litigation.

1. Enter your name in courthouse register.
2. Select your case type and level of difficulty.
3. Select your role either as defendant or prosecutor.
4. Brief narrative describes your case and goal.
5. When called to court, begin your opening argument. If you do things out of order, your associate reminds you of the correct order.
6. Type your opening argument in the space provided.
7. Check your menu of evidence. See what facts you have available.
8. Call your first witness from menu of witnesses. Type in your question on the inquiry board.

FIGURE 3.5 (continued)

9. Type in your closing argument.
10. Await your verdict.
11. Be ready for preprogrammed replies. When you're ready to ask questions again, press mouse and your inquiry board appears.
12. Any time you badger witness, take too much time, or do something wrong, the judge gives you a warning. When you receive two warnings, you automatically get cited for contempt of court and sent to jail. You must return to law school for review of the mistake before starting a new case.

What Developer Can Provide

1. Conceptual blueprint, narrative scenarios, and technical background on case details

2. Introductory software instructions; textual material on litigation history, process, or ethical responsibilities of attorneys; etc.

What Developer Needs from Publisher

1. Computer programmer who can design the code for Macintosh, IBM, etc., operating system

Proposal #2

"My Therapist"

Developers of Idea: Douglas H. Ruben, PhD and Marilyn J. Ruben
Type of Program: Interactive counseling movie, in which you are the therapist
Computer Market: Macintosh, IBM, etc.

Brief Summary

"My Therapist" is a thrilling adventure into the mysterious world of human behavior. Take apart what people do in easy-to-understand ways that put users in the therapist's seat on giving advice on personal issues. Choose the type of problem from the diagnosis menu (e.g., anxiety, depression, substance abuse, marriage, family) and level of difficulty: Beginner (quit cigarette smoking, lose weight, etc.), Intermediate (parent-child problems, phobia, etc.) or Advanced (chronic anxiety, substance abuse, etc.). Welcome your male or female child, adolescent, or adult client to the session.

Start off your first interview using the diagnosis template, which helps users organize questions about history, presenting problem, and types of therapy (individual, family, marriage). Now comes the fun part. Therapy sessions consist of three parts: (a) questions/answers, (b) techniques, and (c) homework assignments. For every question there are many preprogrammed answers. How do you analyze them? You guess.

Don't rely on guesswork; check the THEY MEAN menu (e.g., "I'm angry" = person is angry, "Drinking makes me feel good" = person is alcoholic, "I want people to like me" = person hates rejection). Now choose from strategy menu (e.g., relaxation, assertiveness, change thinking). Last, you're ready to choose from the homework menu (every day, once a day, get medication, get a labotomy, get electro-convulsive therapy (ECT), get another therapist, get a physical exam, etc.).

Type your question on the Inquiry Board and be ready for all sorts of hoops. What if your client cries, threatens suicide, homicide, verbally or physically threatens you, is property destructive, is silent and says nothing, or simply leaves the office? Check the menu of quick-fixes to remedy the situation (call police, end session, etc.).

When conducting sessions, if you say the wrong thing or make the wrong analysis, your associate watching through a two-way mirror will signal you with a warning message on the screen. Two warnings and it's too late; the person kills himself, kills another person, or sues you.

Basic Steps

Conceptually, this game proceeds in the following sequential order:

FIGURE 3.5 (continued)

First, you attend "Counseling School" for briefing. Then, begin your session.

1. Your secretary asks that you select your client/problem from the register.
2. Select your diagnosis and level of difficulty.
3. Brief narrative describes background on client.
4. If it's the first session with client, begin your interview using the diagnostic template. Subsequent sessions start with questions/answers.
5. Begin questions/answers. Write questions on the Inquiry Board. If you say or do the wrong thing or in the wrong order, your associate reminds you of the correct order. On the second warning, something bad happens.
6. Be ready for preprogrammed replies. When you're ready to ask questions again, just press the mouse and your inquiry board appears.
7. Read client replies, then check THEY MEAN menu. Continue questions.
8. When ready for strategy, choose strategy from menu. Again, your associate might stop you with a warning.
9. Now choose from the homework menu.
10. Any time you receive two warnings you automatically lose your client or he is taken over by your associate. Then you must return to counseling school for review of the mistake before selecting a new client.

What Developer Can Provide

1. Conceptual blueprint, narrative scenarios, and technical background on case details

2. Introductory software instructions, textual material on history of psychotherapy and type of therapies used in game, process or ethical responsibilities of counselors, etc.

What Developer Needs from Publisher

1. Computer programmer who can design the code for Macintosh, IBM, etc. operating system

The last section, *What developers need from publishers,* is usually the same. You want a computer programmer whose training is versatile enough to engineer your ideas for both Macintosh and IBM models.

What's the Best Form of Communication?

Software publishers are on the cutting edge of technocivilization. They are frequently programmers themselves attuned to the stiff market rivalry of software products and very picky about what they choose. They may spend most of the day in front of a computer debugging a program or creatively inventing new sequences. They are in the trenches getting dirty and constantly switching back and forth from administrator to technical analyst. They usually operate small shops, with few staff and low overhead. But in-house production only comprises a fraction of their output. Ideas from the outside are invited, especially from experts whose paradigms for software are fabulously original, marketable, and simple to write.

Knowing they are impossible to reach, make your first contact either through facsimile or e-mail. Fax an inquiry letter with or without the proposal to wave down the publisher. Simultaneously send a follow-up e-mail elaborating on your idea and willingness to work with his or her programming staff, for example, at a reduced royalty rate. Table 3.3 reviews other pros and cons of communication modes. Note, in general, that phone calls or snail mail are doomed to fail. They rarely reach your target reader. E-mail is at least within the publisher's natural habitat (e.g., his or her computer) and convincingly proves that you are computer literate and may have instincts on what works in an entertaining software program.

VIDEO, TV, AND INFOMERCIAL PROPOSALS

Revenues can be sizable in the video and TV business. In Chapter 6 the trends in this business and how to outsmart veteran scriptwriters for a piece of the dollar action are discussed in detail. For now, let's consider the three styles of submissions likely to stimu-

TABLE 3.3. Advantages and disadvantages of communication media for software proposal

Type of Media	Advantages	Disadvantages
Snail mail	Attachments sent along. Logic of program explained. Your background explained. Credibility on stationery.	Too long to arrive. Information overload for editor. Slow editorial reply. Gives editor reason to ignore it.
Fax	Persuasive pitch. Invites immediate dialogue. Taps "impulsive" industry.	Limits documents sent. One chance for perfect pitch.
E-mail	Shows use of technology. Casual, softer approach. Fast editorial reply.	Limited space for attachments. No graphic capabilities. Pitch may be less credible.
Phone call	Piques temporary interest. Fast invite to send details.	Might not reach editors. Might not reach programmers. Need to send letter, fax, or e-mail anyway.

late a producer's attention. These are *news releases, summaries,* and *lists of program ideas.*

A news release is a style of inquiry letter usually sent by fax, which opens with a headline of "For Producers Only," followed by a logline resembling a feature news story (see Figure 3.6). Write the paragraph as if typed by a reporter. Compose it in a fast-moving, easy-to-read style. Instantly hit the reader between the eyes with riveting cliffhangers and a highly charged threat of controversy. Note where it reads "560 kilograms of uranium more explosive than ten times the bombs dropped on Hiroshima and Nagasaki combined." This stimulates intrigue in most readers who are shocked, fascinated, and lured into questioning the details further.

Begin the letter with a generic address to "producer" and identify in three paragraphs the story line and purpose of contacting the producer. Save the last paragraph for instructions on how to be

FIGURE 3.6. Cover letter to motion picture producer for proposal to make movie from published book

BEST IMPRESSIONS INTERNATIONAL INCORPORATED

4211 OKEMOS ROAD, SUITE 22, OKEMOS, MICHIGAN 48864, U.S.A.
FAX or PHONE: 517-347-0944; PHONE: 1-800-595-BEST; local 347-1811

FOR PRODUCERS ONLY

Salt Lake City, Utah– *Shocking proof of Germany's WWII atomic weapons sold to Japan! 560 kilograms of uranium more explosive than ten times the bombs dropped on Hiroshima and Nagasaki combined. Secretly shipped to Japan, it never got there. And we know why. This incredibly heroic story of the aborted U-boat voyage is based on U.S. and German classified documents, is in press, and is titled* **Hitler's Revenge**. *It's waiting for you to bring it to the screen.*

Dear Producer:

This is more than history. Astounding evidence documents that Germany not only had powerful atomic know-how, but get this: their experts and materials did Americans a favor. They finished off the bombs, ending war in the Pacific. Can't believe it? There's more. Find out when you read a prepublication copy of **Hitler's Revenge.**

Hitler's Revenge is a chilling account of how SS officers escaped by plane to Argentina, how Hitler's body couldn't possibly be incinerated, and how a revamped U-boat bound for Japan surrendered at the last moment.

We invite you to consider this property for production. It's perfect for a documentary or full-length motion picture. Attached is a synopsis for starters. The book will be adapted to screenplay/teleplay by D. RUBEN.

WANT TO REACH US TODAY? E-mail us at mjruben@aol.com, or fax us at 517-347-0944. We look forward to hearing from you soon.

Cordially,

Doug Ruben

P.S. Since we produce TV shows such as *The Celebrity Golf Show*, but are looking to break into feature films, we'd be happy to coproduce and handle locations or arrangements in the United States.

reached day or night. Include in this paragraph or as a postscript any other similar video projects in your repertoire, which you feel can contribute to the producer's decision.

A *summary* is a one-page synopsis of the script, book, or other idea proposed for video adaptation (see Figure 3.7). For documentaries, for example, point out in the first paragraph the biographical story line or vantage point and data collection system. In Figure 3.7, we see the protagonist is an amateur historian who stumbles across odd details while reading for pleasure. Coupled with his own memory of wartime experiences, he vigilantly searches governmental archives and uses the Freedom of Information (FOI) system to retrieve declassified documents.

A *list* is used primarily for direct response TV pitches (see Figure 3.8). There are several ways to propose an infomerical, one of which appeared in Chapter 1 of *Publicity for Mental Health Clinicians*. Alternatively, you can take the easier route of listing power titles followed by a description of the proposed product. In a cover letter explain your scriptwriting or self-help, how-to writing experiences, ability to write under pressure and do rewrites, and willingness to travel on-site for filming. As most infomercial scribing is done in house, breaking into the industry requires a showstopping idea ingeniously able to attract a strong market for late and early morning airings. Figure 3.8 illustrates some bizarre titles for sensationalistic shows that, with the right scripting and product development, can rake in millions for the South American and Mexican shopping channels.

What's the Best Form of Communication?

The trouble with reaching industrial video, TV, and infomercial producers is that if they are still in business, they are on location shooting a film. Communication either waits until they return or is forwarded by facsimile. Table 3.4 offers thoughts on advantages versus disadvantages on how to reach producers. However, the surest way to stop a producer in his or her tracks is by e-mail or fax. Today directors, producers, and most above-the-line staff (administrators and talent) carry portable computers with fax-modem capabilities. They plug them in at hotels and will send or retrieve e-mail messages at night or before arriving on the set in the morning.

FIGURE 3.7. Proposal for teleplay or screenplay

Hitler's Revenge

By Arthur Naujoks and Doug Ruben
For teleplay or screenplay
Story by Arthur Naujoks, screenplay by Doug Ruben

The story begins with first-person character revealing that he was a German soldier who stumbled across information that piqued his curiosity. He asked questions of friends, even asked a neighbor who was on the flight crew of atom-bomb drop on Nagasaki about what this "uranium" stuff was. Obsessed with intrigue, he sent Freedom of Information (FOI) requests to the Federal Government hoping for answers. Replies from Capitol Hill disturbed him, with documents reporting what looked like a coverup, that is, a conspiracy involving Japan and Germany over development and warfare use of the atom bomb. From his notes and thumbing through articles and documents a pattern emerges. The rest of the book unfolds this pattern piece by piece, until we learn why the pieces are so important to our German soldier. Here are the pieces he finds:

Documented chronicles are uncovered of German atomic research in 1938 with Otto Hahn splitting the atom and primarily Jewish scientists exploring atomic fission. As the Fuhrer rose to power, Einstein, Oppenheimer, Teller, and Meitner, among others, fled Germany, leaving notebooks on how to experimentally synthesize uranium minerals into a compound called Isotope-U235. Germany's surplus of raw uranium made it possible to amass large quantities to extract atoms, predating America's Manhattan project. Even Britain's destruction of the Norwegian heavy water plant, celebrated as ending German research, in truth did not do any damage.

But research became static, while mutiny among Hitler's closest generals in 1944 resulted in a failed assassination attempt. Realizing his days were numbered, Hitler unveiled an incredible solution to his defeat. First, he secretly arranged for shipments of his booties to Argentina by entrusting the unscrupulous Evita Peron, then Evita Duarte, to open four bank accounts. Into each account were liquidated assets from the gold, silver, and other priceless jewels of prisoners and corpses. Orders from General Bormann called for two U-boats with precious cargo to proceed to Cadez, Spain, then onward to Argentina. Unsuspecting shipments made their way through turbulent waters. But these precautionary steps were only a prelude to the northern escape route.

Hitler masterminded an Alcatraz-like escape more daring than Houdini's magic. He dispatched an emergency call for his confidant female aviator, Hanna Reitsch. Historically reconstructing the final hours, Hitler and Eva Braun left his bunker before the Russian army arrived, quickly joining Reitsch on the monoplane. The plane took off under radar on a boulevard and landed at Reschlin Airport, north of Berlin.

FIGURE 3.7 (continued)

From there he flew to the Norway harbor at Christiansand, ready to board the U-234. Early en route, the U-234 had a rendezvous with another ship. Log records show that 12 crew mysteriously disembarked the U-234 and boarded the other vessel. Hitler and his entourage may have been among them.

In his last act as Nazi Fuhrer, Hitler ordered a meeting with Japan ambassador Oshima to conspire to purchase uranium and extract isotope U-235 in return for his safe passage. Loaded carefully into gold-insulated cylinders were highly radioactive compounds (560 kilograms of uranium) together with an advanced arsenal. Japan was to build the triumphant atomic destruction machine. Recorded accounts of the U-234 crew after Hitler supposedly escaped to sanctuary are both baffling and miraculous. Naval commander Fehler introspectively reconsidered his mission; he consulted, first, his friend Karl Pfaff before asking General Kessler to detour from Japan into northern waters where they would rendezvous with American forces. When word of this surrender reached cargo supervisors Oberst Shoji and Fregatten-Kapitain Tomonaga, both from the Japanese Imperial Army, rather than suffer humiliation, they upheld their honor and committed suicide.

Safely reaching the allies, the skipper surrendered his vessel 500 miles south of Newfoundland to the U.S. Destroyer *Sutton*. The enormous size of this captured German vessel and its prize-winning cargo was unbelievable. More startling, however, is that from classified interrogation records can be found General Kessler's agreement to help end the war in the Pacific. Teamed again with their German cohorts, atomic scientists put the final touches on fissionable uranium as a heat-propelled explosive nightmare. In fact, German technology helped build the destructive death-bomb that backfired on Japan, the very nation who months earlier would have executed Hitler's revenge and caused Armageddon.

FIGURE 3.8. Proposal for infomercials

BEST IMPRESSIONS INTERNATIONAL INCORPORATED

4211 OKEMOS ROAD, SUITE 22, OKEMOS, MICHIGAN 48864, U.S.A.
FAX or PHONE: 517-347-0944; PHONE: 1-800-595-BEST; local 347-1811

Program Ideas for Infomercials for South American/Mexican Markets or for New Shopping Channel

Program Titles

1. **Power Speak!** Program for English as Second Language
2. **Megamarket Your Skills!** One-minute methods for rapid self-motivation and financial freedom through marketing one's trades, skills, and talents
3. **Super Secrets to Success!** One-minute methods to escape depression, feel upbeat, motivated, and take initiative
4. **Color Me Beautiful!** Cosmetic program (like Victoria Principal's package) for wealthy-looking skin on a working woman's budget
5. **Smoker Stopper.** Use of highly effective mind-altering methods to stop smoking overnight without withdrawal, cravings, or relapse. (Infomercial already finished/owned by Best Impressions, or, can do new one)
6. **Maximum Sexual Control.** Program showing easy steps for daily sexual enhancement and rapid solutions to sexual hangups
7. **Ultra-Body Builder.** 30-day bodybuilding workout program using home aerobics, simple calisthenics, and weight lifting without expensive or heavy equipment
8. **Psychic Love Connection.** Personalized horoscope predicting the perfect mate, where and how to love, and other romantic expectations
9. **Pet Astrology.** Yes, it sounds funny, but we'll be the first on the block to offer this blockbuster product. Obtain horoscope of your pet based on month of birth, tied into owner's month of birth, to predict which dogs should go with which owners, which dogs should breed together, best food to feed your pet, and so forth.

Products

1. Audiocassette program (three to four tapes)
2. Booklet
3. Software (if PC computers are popular)

TABLE 3.4. Advantages and Disadvantages of Communication Media for Video and TV Proposals

Type of Media	Advantages	Disadvantages
Snail mail	Video plot fully explained. Attachments sent. Will be read by producer.	Too amateur. Slow producer reply. High rejection rate.
Fax	Read instantly and replied to. Pitch briefer, simpler. Preferred mode for response.	May be rerouted or lost. If rejected, then ignored.
E-mail Phone-call	Reach producer at home. Pitch idea that moment. Friendly, softer, less wait.	Rarely read or logged on to. Risk of interruption or rude rejection.

I recall, for instance, when filming *The Celebrity Golf Show* in Palm Springs, California, I would seize early morning hours logging onto my internet server to check my e-mail messages. Or, I would correspond by fax back to Michigan. No other time was set aside for reading mail or answering phone calls.

CONSTRUCTING WEB PAGE PROPOSALS

For advertising your web services, there are multiple formats currently in vogue. But one thing needs to be clear. Website construction is neither for publishers nor editors. It is a purely entrepreneurial business where you target the buyers and use direct marketing to reach them (Prima, 1996). You are in total control. You can buy customer mailing lists or generate them entirely on your own, usually from published lists of local, state, or regional businesses. Creating your own web shop is different in that you are not asking another agency to materialize your idea. That's what publishers or producers do. You are the founder and implementer of all the ideas invested in web development. It's your baby.

Website buyers may or may not know what the internet and world wide web actually are. Informed buyers need little persuasion other than convincing them that your graphic artistry will produce a high number of "hits" (visits by readers). Uninformed buyers may be skeptical of cyberspace and look to you for compassion, guidance, and education. That accounts for two different types of proposals: *web training* and *web construction.*

Web Training

Advertisements that directly focus on computer illiterates are offering on-line consulting and training on internet access, server selections, and website research. Letters look more like announcements, alerting net browsers, retailers, or any customer to a more efficient superhighway through your advice. Acting like strategically placed gasoline stations along the interstate, you are available as a "help file" at any point where the net-browsing motorist conks out and needs repair. After giving directions or fueling them with suggestions, they go on their merry way until a later time when they are again on empty.

Charges for on-line consultation vary by "contact minute" or "per site contact." Contact minutes are charged at $1.99 to $3.00 a minute, similar to what it costs for a 900 number. Costs for "per site contact" may vary from $3.00 to $6.00. Billing is usually done monthly through e-mail with a predesigned form asking for a major credit card.

So, now that you know what to charge and the basic service to offer, *what exactly do you deliver?* Good question. You're a navigator providing up-to-date longitudinal and latitudinal coordinates for the website, chat groups, and other internet playgrounds where customers seek information. For instance, suppose a customer wants life insurance. You might suggest the customer type in the website "http://www.humana.com/," which links him or her up with Humana Health Care plans. This site provides brochures with typical company information, financials, office locations, history, and promising insurance programs.

Suppose, instead, the person wants to buy a unique gift for a loved one. Fine, you say—on to Neiman Marcus ("http://www.neimanmarcus.com/). Or say the person hates to smudge fingers on newsprint. Offer on-line reading of *The New York Times* (http://www.nytimes.com/info/contents/textpath.html).

Constant upgrades and new site listings fill the spectrum of possible web page referrals. For tabloid-hungry buyers, place an asterick in your web portfolio next to sex and UFO sites. Both get thousands of hits (visitors) and surge you through multimedia trips in cyberspace. Sex sites, for example, cover dating services, sex chat sessions, tips for safe sex, and cruising cyber bars. But don't take my word for it. Check out Candyland (http://www.candyland.com/net), Clublove (http://www.adultplayground.com/oa), and uncensored adult services (http://www.onalt.com).

In UFO circles, sample a close encounter of your own with extraterrestrials (http://www.io.org/dnewton/ufo.html). Read firsthand confessions by alien abductees on experiments done on humans (http://www.ee.fit.edu/users/lpinto/sec-abd.html OR http://tucson.com/ufotest/). Or, receive recent reports of sightings, updates on crop circles, and other research phenomena from the Mutual UFO Network website (MUFON) (http://www.rutgers.edu/-mcgrew/mufon).

You can find this spectrum of sites ahead of time in several ways. First is by subscribing to or buying at the newsstand several PC computer and internet magazines. Each magazine usually highlights new website pages with complete listings of the Uniform Resource Location (URL) addresses. Top-ranked computer magazines supplying updated facts, figures, and consumer tips for online servers and internet access are listed in Table 3.5.

Second, you can use the "search engines" or indexes already built into the internet, which enable web users to search for sites using keywords. The most popular one is *Yahoo* (http://www.yahoo.com/). This one-time simple directory invented by two college students has earned them millions in sales to other companies wanting advertising space on their highly frequented service. For example, Yahoo recently landed a deal with Gannett Broadcasting Corporation for joint promotion of each other's content. Yahoo will feature more news stories from the Gannett's syndicates of ABC and CBS stations while Gannett will sell advertising space for Yahoo. A sweet deal, to say the least.

TABLE 3.5. Top-ranked computer magazines

The Net
phone: 416-696-1661
fax: 415-696-1678
e-mail: subscribe@thenet-usa.com
$45.95/yr.

PC Gamer
phone: 800-706-9500
$47.95/yr

Next Generation
phone: 800-706-9500
e-mail: NGSUBS@aol.com
$29/yr

NetGuide
phone: 800-829-0421
fax: 516-562-7406
e-mail: crenta@cmp.com
$22.97/yr

Online Access
phone: 800-36-MODEM
e-mail: 74514.3363@compuserve.com
$41.95/yr

Users of Yahoo, called *yahooligans,* find this browser fun and easy. While less popular, other search engines at your fingertips include Lycos, Infoseek, Webcrawler, Alta Vista, and WWWWorm.

Lycos (http://www. lycos.com) is easily searchable by keywords and provides matches to each word with list sites. Infoseek (http://www2.infoseek.com) offers a paid service in which you get an extensive search. Webcrawler (http://webcrawler.com) lets you type in your keywords, choose what you want, and enables you to choose the results you want displayed. Alta Vista (http://www.alta-vista.digital.com) is a new entry offering a "super spider" tool. Creators at Digital Equipment say it makes searches faster and more precisely. Searches cover an exhaustive 16 million pages in a data-base. WWWWorm (http://www.cs.colorado.edu/mcbryan/www.com) focuses on keyword searches but is limited as a browser. Depth of its coverage may be inferior to other search tools.

Web Construction

The other mechanism for web consulting is to build a web page and offer linking services (see Figure 3.9).

The inquiry letter is a generic form sent by mail order or unsolic-ited e-mail to multiple customers who you believe are prime buyers. It is a two-page document opening with a pulsating headline and brief description on how the service works. Figure 3.9 combines both features in one document. It describes a linking service where-upon buyers with existing products can place their ad or link their ad (if they have web pages) to a central website. This web-connect page acts as an outlet mall with many vendors renting space. A "hit" on their page would link the curious shopper directly to their goods and services either on the page we provide or to the vendor's own page.

On the second page, it requests that they contact us for more information on website construction. Why? Because the costs will vary. If they want a subsite to our main web page, the price may be $300 to $500, depending on multimedia graphics used. If, on the other hand, they want a freestanding web page independent of our own web page and linked up with other web sites, costs can run as high as $10,000.

Web page construction demands a high price tag since the artistry and programming are technically complex (Behram, 1995; Magid, Matthews and Jones, 1995; Morris, 1996; Prevost and McArdle, 1996; Stross, 1996). Simpler website construction programs, how-ever, are hitting the department stores and may tempt consumers to do website development themselves. Self-generated web pages using user-friendly graphic programs are fast and instantly turn you into a homegrown webmaster. Table 3.6 gives you a sample of affordable web construction software sold at most department stores. Try these

FIGURE 3.9. Advertisement for website construction

BEST IMPRESSIONS INTERNATIONAL INCORPORATED

4211 OKEMOS ROAD, SUITE 22, OKEMOS, MICHIGAN 48864, U.S.A.
PHONE or FAX: 517-347-0944; PHONE: 1-800-595-BEST

Should your product be seen by 30 million buyers?

WEB-Connect today.

Imagine showing your product at a 24-hour continuous trade show. Combine that with the lightening speed of today's internet magic and you have WEB-Connect. Web Connect is your fastest marketing strategy for worldwide consumers. It allows you, the product owner or manufacturer, to place your product ad on Best Impressions International's WEB-HOME pages for immediate buyer access. Marketing on the Web (World Wide Web) is easy, reliable, and costs a fraction of what it costs to run advertisements on TV, radio, or newspapers. Advertising on WEB-Connect boosts you into the tech-age generation of sophisticated, affluent buyers surfing cyberspace for the best product around.

What you need for Web-Connect

To be announced soon are home-pages or "web pages" owned and operated by Best Impressions International Inc. Pages are like large highway billboards able to be viewed by over 30 million subscribers to different internet vendor services. For your advertisement, you need the following:

- Products (100+ volume or easy access to this amount)
- 1-800 number or use of our partial fulfillment process
- Capability to ship the product to the buyer

How does it work?

You rent space on the web page. As web readers open the web page, they see the advertisers. Once a person reads your logline, for example, "High-tech space toys for kids," he or she clicks twice on your logline and it opens a separate page listing your products and costs. Your page can be graphic, audio, or possibly even video. It's multimedia. That page also gives directions on how to order the products. Customers can call your 1-800 number directly where they can e-mail their order to our computer where we process the order and charge it to VISA or MASTERCARD, and in

FIGURE 3.9 (continued)

turn give the order and payment to you. But here's the best part. The way worldwide viewers know that your ad exists is by *links*. Think of links as a subway. You get from one web page to another web page by links. And *very fast*. The more web pages we pay to have our page linked with, the more people know to check your ad out.

What does it cost?

There are four costs: first, set-up costs; second, monthly rental costs; third, link costs; and fourth, partial fulfillment costs. Final costs will be available in a month. For now, here are the current costs we know about:

Set-Up Cost:	$250
Monthly Rental Cost:	to be announced ($50 to $150)
Link Cost:	$15 per link site (may change)
Partial Fulfillment Cost:	15% of the per unit product order, which pays for

  • processing the order.
  • checking out VISA/MASTERCARD orders.
  • communicating your order.
  • sending you balance of payment.
  For instance, if product sells for $8.00 + $2.00 shipping and handling, we get $1.50 (15% of $10.00).

Any other services you provide on WEB?

Sure do. Ask us about how we can set up your own web page. We would be happy to give you more details and quote you prices. It's a lot more effort on your part, but has many advantages as well.

HOW DO I GET STARTED?

Give us a call and we'll set you up with a full package program to get you on-line with the fastest growing medium for advertising.

software helpers to get a feel of the action. When you're comfortable with them, experiment with color, graphics, and design tips for creating a killer website (e.g., Cooper, 1996).

Websites also are available through popular on-line servers such as Prodigy and America Online. Servers now offer subscribers a free, easy-to-load web page (Bankston, 1995; Gray, 1996; Townsend, 1996; Sosinsky, 1995; Withers, 1995).

Which Server to Use?

How do you get from a PC to an on-line service? Simple. It's called a modem. Modem speeds of 1200 bps (bytes per second), 2400 BPS, 14.4 BPS or 28.8 BPS all enable data transmission from your computer through the telephone line to vast networks worldwide. Access to each network begins by logging in with a password or special code, much like activating or deactivating an alarm. Passwords and codes activate a connection to the server, where you are identified as a paid subscriber and eligible for admission. Once logged on, you can click your mouse on any number of icons that open message boards, information centers, advertisements, interactive games, or the internet. On-line subscriber networks make your surfing easy. They even provide a searching device that allows you to type in a subject's key words and get transferred to it immediately.

Is one on-line service better than another? Not really. Experts argue pros and cons for each of the four major national and international online services: Compuserve, America Online, Prodigy, and Microsoft Network. Table 3.7 overviews subscription information for each of these commercial on-line users.

America Online (AOL), the premiere service, enjoys a commanding lead in international coverage. Recently expanded to Great Britain and Germany, AOL's speedway provides fast, mouse-friendly navigation around its thousands of forums, newsgroups, and informational hot spots. It is geared to adults in their twenties and thirties. Log-on simplicity is good for on-line beginners since it has step-by-step screen instructions. Psychology, scriptwriting, book writing, and several entertainment sites round out its venues for visiting. Even on slow modem speeds (1200 bps), movement in AOL is fine for casual Sunday drivers. For impatient researchers,

TABLE 3.6. Web construction software programs

Software	Requires	Price	Contact
All-in-one page surfing and publishing kit	Windows Windows 95	$79.99	The Coriolis Group 800-410-0192
Asymetrix Web 3D	Windows Windows 95	$69.96	Microwarehouse (distributor) 800-367-7080
Backstage Desktop Studio	Windows Windows 95	$499.95	Microwarehouse (distributor) 800-367-7080
Incontext Spider 1.1	Windows Windows 95	$99	InContext Systems 800-263-0127
PageMill 1.0	Windows Windows 95	$149	Adobe Systems 800-642-3623
3-D Website Builder	Windows Windows 95	$99.95	Microwarehouse (distributor) 800-367-7080
Web Buddy	Windows Windows 95	$49.95	Microwarehouse (distributor) 800-367-7080
WebWizard	Windows Windows 95	$10	ARTA Media Group http://www.halcy-on.com/artamedia /webwizard

TABLE 3.7. Subscription information for major commercial on-line services

Name of Service	Sign-Up Number	Price Structure
America Online	800-827-6364	$19.95/month for unlimited access.
Compuserve	800-848-8990	$9.95/month includes 5 hours free + $2.95 for each additional hour. Or $24.95/month includes 20 free hours +$1.95 for each additional hour.
Prodigy	800-776-3449	$9.95/month includes 5 hours free + $2.95 for each additional hour. Or $29.95/month includes 30 free hours +$2.95 for each additional hour.
Microsoft Network	http://www.msn.com/msn.htm	$4.95/month includes 3 hours free + $2.50 for each additional hour. Or $19.95/month includes 20 free hours + $2.00 for each additional hour.

you may find any modem speed less than 28.8 bps unbearable. A second drawback is its limited internet access. AOL's web browser, or function for viewing websites, is slow to load artwork and jump to new websites. Its snail's pace can be incredibly frustrating for jetsetters accustomed to browsing speeds of, for example, Netscape.

Compuserve offers news, weather, sports, and shopping, plus hundreds of á la carte chat rooms and forums. Traditionally, it has been marketed as a family service. Most users are male Caucasians, ages 30 to 50, affluent, and experienced with computers. Services tend to cater to business-minded users. Extra costs apply to file libraries with downloadable documents, access to the internet, and use of special databases such as Showbiz Forum. Flexibility is a big plus for Compuserve's less-graphic formats and user-friendly interfaces. On the downside, internet access is difficult and requires you to work a little harder than you would on other services.

Prodigy is colorful, personable, and like AOL, geared toward families with children. Hailed as the first on-line service to offer web access, Prodigy's maturity suffered a setback when it overdosed users with a jungle of graphics. Unless modem speeds well exceed 14.4 bps, loading web pages can take forever. Personally, I found Prodigy still addicted to DOS-like format and less conducive to mouse commands.

Microsoft Network is Bill Gates' brainchild. The hoopla surrounding its release with Windows 95 stemmed more from political rivalry than technologic fears. Compared to other services, logging on is quite facile. The sign-up sequence, welcome page, and graphic navigational system begin on the desktop with an icon that users need only double-click with the mouse. Connectivity is fast, unencumbered by graphic forestry, and allows for complete internet access. So, what's wrong with it? Apart from horror stories about installation of Windows 95, the biggest pitfall is e-mail restriction. Users can only send e-mail to readers within its Microsoft exchange rather than across any on-line service including the internet.

Web Links

Even a good on-line service and a good web page won't guarantee sales. Self-made web pages need a link. You can be a specialist in purely linking up web sites with other site connections, just as if the customer appeared in multiple Yellow Page directories. Links allow visitors to jump from a contracted site to the customer's site, providing the customer with an increased amount of targeted visitors (or "hits"). It is a surefire way to capitalize on the congested internet traffic for maximum exposure of your customer's product. Real estate entrepreneurs have been doing it for months. For example, *Property-Link* (http://www.property-link.com) helps brokers and landlords reach worldwide audiences either by hooking them to your website or by featuring your property in mass e-mail marketing.

What do you charge them? It varies. Most linking fees are about $25 per link per month. Actual pricing is determined by the site owners, or the websites onto which you link your customer's web page. Some may generously allow you to link it for free, while others charge a premium for their space. In addition, charge a one-time setup fee of $30 per link per site, and ask for a minimum link charge of $75 per month. Will these prices gouge the customer and discourage their utilization of your service? No, not at all. Even if these prices sound hefty, realize that conventional paper advertising costs double or triple the amount for on-line links. A display ad run in the Yellow Pages, for example, is $2,500 per year, averaging out to $200 per month. And that's only for one directory targeting one regional area. Compare that to $75 per month plus, say, two links at $25 for a total monthly cost of $125. For these dollars you reach 30 million potential buyers worldwide. I think it's a better deal, don't you?

What's the Best Form of Communication?

Companies or individuals planning on enlarging their computer capacities already are on-line and have past first grade in cyberschool. They are voraciously hungry and anxious to eat their way through the chocolate factory of worldwide buyers. They know buyers exist, they realize they have salable products, and now look for brokers who can be matchmakers between their hopes and dreams. You can reach these parties best by e-mailing them. While facsimiles may also catch their attention, I recommend you use the mode of communication you plan on helping your customer with:

namely, the computer. Table 3.8 further identifies the advantages and disadvantages of e-mail versus other means of customer contact.

TABLE 3.8. Advantages and disadvantages of communication media for constructing web page proposals

Type of Media	Advantages	Disadvantages
Snail mail	Attach samples. Describe design ideas.	Most pitches done electronically. Doesn't show computer literacy.
Fax	Fast reply. Stimulates interest. Solicits phone call or e-mail.	Poor transmission quality for attachments.
E-mail	Guarantee buyer contact. Shows use of technology. Files sent in attachments. Faster buyer replies.	Quality of attachments lost. Limited multimedia samples sent. Buyer may distrust credentials.
Phone call	Pitch gets you in the door. Forces brevity.	Work samples absent. Follow through must be fast, like overnight.

GHOSTWRITING AND EDITING PROPOSALS

Today, ghostwriters are the secret force behind power engine authors. Celebrity biographies, in particular, are fertile ground for freelancers able to interview effectively, and generate story line mixed with the right chemistry of personality and controversy. Then they spit it out neatly on a dish for publishers. Ghostwriting services consequently have picked up steam over the past five years, opening doors for nonjournalists and nontraditional scriptdoctors. Now, writing experts from any discipline, presuming they are flexible and marketable, can be the invisible scribe for best-selling trade books and magazine articles.

Proposals are usually not formal nor directly solicitive but more in response to an editor's referrals or author requests. Editor's referrals occur when publishing houses have too few editors to handle the influx of manuscript copyediting or when authors under contract turn in lousy products. When this happens, editors look outside to reliable freelancers who can offset their load. Another editor referral occurs when authors telephone in ambitious ideas but are inexperienced writers and need assistance with manuscript structure or, plainly, they need somebody *to write their ideas for them.* Referrals given by the editor are easy to follow up with a phone call or snail mail.

A second source of ghostwriting and editing contacts is through cold calls. Sure, you can run a display ad in writing magazines and even plot a direct-mail campaign targeting young, unseasoned writers, but there is a nasty side effect of this approach: advertising costs. Mailing lists cost hundreds upon hundreds of dollars and you receive a "lick and a promise" guarantee whether the list is new, old, hot, or cold. Cold lists, of course, would be dead-end recipients who toss out your unsolicited mail. The same outcome is nearly certain for display ads. Graphically attractive ads, on average, generate 5 to 10 percent response rate if the means of responding is cheap, quick, and effortless. For example, if readers can phone in questions on your 800 number, expect a higher response rate. Calls made long distance will kill your response rate. Overall, expenditures for that display ad, 800 number, and manpower to answer the 800 line (unless you have super voice mail) are painfully high.

Alternatively, use the e-mail system. In user lists or bulletin boards where authors are openly asking for ghostwriters, editors, or helpers, send an e-mail to them describing your service. For example, America Online offers the "Writer's Club," in which different categories from fiction, nonfiction, scriptwriting, and so forth include author exchanges, commercial services, and a fishbowl of new clients. Design your e-mail to be friendly and to the point (see Figure 3.10). Include in it your basic services, why you or your agency has credibility, and how the author may reach you quickly.

Ghostwriting bites are rewarding and can launch a new career within a year. Still, for most authors, trusting a ghostwriter is difficult. Dedicated authors who attend conferences and avidly read trade magazines have heard many horror stories. What horror stories, you ask? They vary. The scariest is when freelance writers

FIGURE 3.10. Ghostwriter and editor solicitation letter for e-mail

GHOSTWRITER

EDITOR

YOUR ONE-STOP BOOK COMPLETION SHOP

FREELANCER WITH INCREDIBLE RECORD

If you are an author, book publisher, or packager wanting fast results from a seasoned professional, try the SCRIPTDOCTOR and MEDIA SERVICES of Best Impressions International Inc.

We are authors who take manuscripts from start to finish. Scriptdoctors of over 40 books and 100 articles successfully helped NEW writers of nonfiction and fiction get PUBLISHED. We write it, edit it, revise it, and even help sell it.

MAKE IT HAPPEN. FIND OUT MORE about our editorial, ghostwriting, marketing, and literary agency services. E-MAIL mjruben@aol.com or call 1-800-595-BEST (scriptdoctor/media services).

---

promise the universe from scribing to guaranteed publishing of the manuscript. What they deliver, however, if they deliver anything, is far from dreamy. They may bail out after receiving advances of $1,000 to $2,000 or complain that competing assignments prevented them from meeting a promised deadline date.

Don't ever promise what you can't deliver. You'd never falsely promise a patient improvements unless you really knew you could help him or her achieve the improvements. Apply the same philosophy in ghostwriting and editing that you faithfully devote yourself to in clinical therapy.

Suspicion of ghostwriters is also why you may choose a less expensive, more of a "see and be convinced" strategy first. A good start-up service is offering a submission package (see Figures 3.11

and 3.12). Submission packages are a showcase of your talents, are easy to construct, and are absolutely in demand by authors. They consist of the one- to five-page book proposal described earlier for a nonfiction (preferred) book along with a supersales inquiry letter. Offered in addition is an editorial service for *only one chapter.* Which chapter the author chooses is up to him or her. That way, authors have a professional portfolio at their disposal for mass publisher submissions.

I recommend you split up the letters to build up momentum and for authors to "look forward" to receiving your reply. Let the second be more explanatory, including an organized questionnaire for authors to complete with their book information, and of course a form for payment via credit cards.

What's the Best Form of Communication?

As strongly indicated, customer contacts for ghostwriting should entirely be through e-mail. The only exception is when inquiry letters follow up on editor referrals. Phone calls are also acceptable for referrals if the editor already contacted the author explaining your service and promising you'd be calling the author soon. Table 3.9 reminds you of the pros and cons of communications routes for ghostwriting and editorial services.

Regulations Governing Unsolicited Electronic Mail

Several times I have mentioned using a mass, unsolicited electronic mailing to target potential customers. Companies of all sizes do this all the time and compete in cyberspace for consumer buyers. Lately, the Direct Marketing Association put the clamp on unlimited advertising with guidelines for cyberspace marketing. These include that marketers do the following:

1. Exercise responsibility and responsiveness to consumers.
2. Post privacy policy on-line.
3. Explain how information is collected and used on-line.
4. Provide consumers the opportunity to opt out.
5. Respect discussion groups that ban commercial intrusion.
6. Be especially sensitive when marketing to children.

FIGURE 3.11. Submission package solicitation letter for e-mail

****
Congratulations on your manuscript!

****

You've finished the hardest part.

Now comes the fun part: You sell it to a publisher. That's right. YOU can do it YOURSELF. All you need is a highly successful SUBMISSION PACKAGE.

SUBMISSION PACKAGES are what publishers want.

Not sure what that is? It's more than an inquiry letter, and it does not involve any of your book chapters. Not at first. What's more, a SUBMISSION PACKAGE rapidly catches the eye of busy publishers. You WILL get a response.

Get a SUBMISSION PACKAGE and beat the competition. Interested in how? Rush a reply to mjruben@aol.com for more details. Or fax us a request at 517-349-1823.

Best Impressions International Inc.

_____

FIGURE 3.12. Submission package follow-up letter for e-mail

****

Thank you for asking about your
SUBMISSION PACKAGES

****

Cheap, fast, and powerfully effective.

A SUBMISSION PACKAGE is a cover letter plus a five- to eight-page "prospectus" or proposal on what your book is about. You describe the topic, special features, table of contents, negotiating angles, marketing angles, and about the authors.

**Now you can have a SUBMISSION PACKAGE prepared for you from the author of over 40 books, including books on publishing, marketing, and promotion.

Cheap, fast, and powerfully effective.

Your personalized SUBMISSION PACKAGE can be yours to send out to publishers for only $200.

An optional service is to have the first chapter of your book edited for only $50. When editors ask for the chapter, you'll have it perfect and ready for them.

All you need to do is fill out the questionnaire below and send your answers by e-mail to mjruben@aol.com or fax it to 517-349-1823. For questions, call 1-800-595-BEST (Ask for scriptdoctor).

QUESTIONNAIRE/ORDER FORM

Below is a series of questions. Please answer each question to the best of your ability. After you have completed the questions, fill out the order form below.

First batch

1. What is the book about?

2. Who will the book appeal to?

3. What genre is the book (e.g., military, self-help)?

4. Why is this the "right time" for the book?

5. What will the book help people to do?

6. What are the main sections of the book?

FIGURE 3.12 (continued)

Second batch

7. How many pages is it?

8. Can you make the script camera (photo) ready?

9. Does it need much editing?

10. When can you realistically finish the editing?

Third batch

11. Can you break your topic down into parts? If so, list the table of contents and subcontents (if you have it).

12. Does your chapter have any real-life examples? Are they listed in the table of contents?

13. Do you have any other important references, notes, graphs, pictures, appendixes, or parts in the chapter you forget in the table of contents?

Fourth batch

14. How is your book better than the competition's?

15. If there is no competition, why will your book be a pioneer?

16. Who is your book for (what audiences)?

17. What can you personally do through your job or connections to publicize the book? How is this better, same, or supplemental to the publisher's promotion?

18. What is it about yourself that makes this book special or will make it a strong contender for high sales?

19. Do you have any TV, radio, or print media interview experience? If so, when, where, on whose show, on what topic?

Fifth batch

20. Can you write a brief biographical paragraph about yourself? Please include what you've published (if anything), your media experience, why you're an expert for this book, and any other outstanding features about yourself.

——— RAPID ORDER FORM ———

Order by phone, e-mail, or fax.

To order by PHONE, call 1-800-595-BEST. Enter mailbox for scriptdoctor. Give name, address, phone number, service wanted, credit card number, (Visa or Mastercard), expiration date, and name on credit card.

By E-MAIL: Fill out the form below and copy/paste this onto a mail-reply to mjruben@aol.com. or fax to 1-517-349-1823.

NAME:

NAME AS APPEARS ON CARD:

ADDRESS:

TELEPHONE #:

CREDIT CARD # (Visa or MC?)

EXPIRATION DATE:

SERVICE WANTED:

      Submission package—$200 _____

First chapter edited—$50 _____

      TOTAL _____

Best Impressions International Inc.

4211 Okemos Road, Suite 22

Okemos, MI 48864

TABLE 3.9. Advantages and disadvantages of communication media for ghost-writing and editing proposals

Type of Media	Advantages	Disadvantages
Snail mail	Shows letterhead. Has personal touch. Can include brochures.	Can get wordy. Can scare off thrifty spenders. Nice materials thrown out.
Fax	Piques interest quickly. Rapid replies given. Shows efficiency.	Older authors may not have fax machines. May give "quick-fix" look. Authors may feel intimidated.
E-mail	Direct, informal, and brief. Reach at home or work. Easy to read, download.	Older authors may not have e-mail. No letterhead glamor. Credibility at first questioned.
Phone call	Personal and friendly. Catharsis for author. Immediate reply.	More therapist than editor. Need follow up in fax, e-mail, or snail mail.

In effect, tapping into electronic networks must now follow regulations cautioning against oversaturation of mail and intrusion of unwanted solicitors. Many customers, for example, hate receiving junk e-mail just as they hate receiving junk snail mail. Now they can stop unsolicited e-mail traffic by following instructions the advertiser posts on his or her e-mail for not receiving future mailings. Guidelines also say "stay out of" bulletin boards, chat groups, or subscriptive news groups where the codified (posted) rules literally ban commercial advertisement. This is not a universal policy for all groups and many even install folders explicitly for advertisers to deposit their goods and services. So, it pays to read the messages of each group's rules before unloading promotional materials.

PROPOSALS TO ACT AS LITERARY AGENT

Observe the same marketing rules when advertising your literary agency services. A literary agent acts to sharpen the manuscript and realistically to find a publishing home for the manuscript. Outlets for publishing vary extensively from traditional royalty houses to subsidy or coventure presses, both of whom may either provide exceptional or destructive ends. Your job in representing the author-client is to (a) recommend what the manuscript needs for a publisher; (b) find the publisher; and (c) negotiate a deal with the publisher, which mutually benefits you and the author (Curtis, 1990; Larsen, 1984).

Unlike ghostwriting, most new authors have completed a manuscript and are now ready for a publisher. They admittedly are deficient in locating the right publisher and are timid about pitching their ideas over the phone. Instead, they look to an authority in the field who is more boldly assertive in telephone conversations and certainly more competent in cultivating a deal for advances, royalties, and sales of subsidiary or secondary book rights. So, authors already want you; you're the bus taking them to their destination. All you have to do is find the right bus stop. And they exist—plenty of them. The richest source of author contacts can be found in on-line writers' groups on Prodigy, America Online, Compuserve, and other leading servers. Internet news groups and websites (found through Yahoo) also are fertile sites, but more difficult to narrow down as to which author needs your services.

Send e-mail announcements that are brief and easy to understand (see Figures 3.13 and 3.14). Follow the protocol of first issuing a teaser inquiry. Even skeptical readers "burned" in previous agency dealings may wonder how you can accomplish these miraculous events. They will request more information, at which time you send your follow-up letter. Details in the follow-up letter cover types of services provided, realistic role of agent and author, and upfront retainer or any other fees expected before or after signing a contract (see Chapter 4).

What's the Best Form of Communication?

Several thousand unpublished authors are target buyers. They either have manuscripts, have ideas for manuscripts, or already had their manuscripts published but are now in the market for publicity, which a literary agency also can provide. Directly corresponding with authors by e-mail can save costly time delays and efficiently reach these eager buyers. Older authors who resist learning computers

FIGURE 3.13. Literary agency letter sent by e-mail

AUTHORS WANTED!

MANUSCRIPTS INVITED!

Fiction, nonfiction, all genres. Fast, on-line response requested. Full literary agency service now expanding on-line with three new services:

 * Rapid publisher search for authors with completed manuscripts.

 * Scriptdoctor (for new authors who need help writing, editing, or polishing book, article, or screenplay)

 * Book marketing (for published authors who need insider tips, leads, and roadmap for promoting their books)

 E-MAIL NOW for more information.

 FOR FAST REPLY ON HOW Best Impressions International Inc. can help you, E-MAIL your book title, brief synopsis, and needs to mjruben@aol.com.

Best Impressions International Inc.

Literary Agency and Production Company

FIGURE 3.14. Literary agency follow-up letter sent by e-mail

Dear Ms. Woods:

Thank you for inquiring about the expanded services at Best Impressions International Inc., your "personal shop" for preparing and publishing books. Your book has very special meaning not only to yourself but to the millions of people literally in your situation who are starving for guidelines on what to do when a person's life is terminal.

At Best Impressions, we have a variety of ways to help mobilize your manuscript from start to finish, from serving as ghostwriter or editorial assistant to literary agent. Prices vary and we would be happy to give you quotes based on your needs. Please see the description of services below. Please contact us soon if we can be of some assistance.

Here's how we can help you at different stages of your manuscript.

* IF YOU HAVE IDEAS BUT HAVE NOT WRITTEN A WORD—

- we will meet with you in person or arrange tape (audio or video) of your story for us to write for you (personal service package).
- we will edit, write from scratch, rewrite, or consult on manuscript revision either before or after finding a publisher.
- we will contact publisher(s), acting as agent and offering the best deal we can find.
- we will offer a marketing component if the publisher does not have one.

* IF YOU HAVE A MANUSCRIPT BUT IT'S BEEN REJECTED—

- we will edit, rewrite, or consult on manuscript revision either before or after finding a publisher. It can be done both ways.
- we will meet with you personally if you want manuscript writing and consultation.
- we will recommend alternate multimedia options for your material if book publishing is not possible.
- we will set up an agency contract with us seeking a publisher for you.

FIGURE 3.14 (continued)

* IF YOU HAVE A PUBLISHED BOOK BUT NEED TO PROMOTE IT—

• we will offer one of three services through our marketing department.

The first is a media package providing insider tips on TV, radio shows, and how to get on media, individualized for your book tours.

The second is a full public relations program in which we set up your tours, media contacts, and act as coordinator.

The third is on-line consulting through AOL or by phone or in person for emergency or troubleshooting problems.

* HOW TO GET STARTED—

1. Send your name, book title, idea, or brief synopsis, and specific service you may need by e-mail to mjruben@aol.com.

2. If you've already done this, send a copy of your manuscript and one-time agency retainer fee of $100 (unless you want a ghostwriter contract), payable to Best Impressions International Inc., to 4211 Okemos Road, Suite 22, Okemos, MI 48864.

3. Within one week, we will send you a contract or give you estimates of services, based on your needs.

PLEASE REPLY IMMEDIATELY SO WE CAN GIVE YOU QUICK FEED-BACK!

Thank you,

Doug Ruben, PhD

President

Best Impressions International Inc.

---

or authors located in rural areas who are unable to dial into local server phone numbers (e.g., netcom) may be inaccessible by e-mail. For them, letter correspondence is the best bet. Consult Table 3.10 for other reasons why one communication modality is better than another.

Even published authors seek literary agents when they are indecisive about which publisher to go with or are entering a new writing discipline. Suddenly, they realize they are out of their league amid the literally millions of diehard scribes sending over-the-transom submissions to publishers on a daily basis. They believe an edge over competition will boost their chances of getting in the door and perceive the literary agent as the gatekeeper to that doorway. Agents know that scholarly writers turned commercial trade authors need coaching guidelines beyond location of a publisher and are potential candidates to purchase multiple agency services.

One way of reaching these changeover authors is by reviewing a publishing company's catalog for books overlapping between lay and academic audiences. Writers of these books may be teetering on the brink of a crossover but may be uncertain what the future holds for them. You can allay their fears by providing security for hesitant authors and discover the absolute bliss of the experience.

TABLE 3.10. Advantages and disadvantages of communication media for acting as literary agent for proposals

Type of Media	Advantages	Disadvantages
Snail mail	Impresses with letterhead. Moves authors at their pace. Printed letter will be read.	Slow and unreliable reply. Easily discarded. Process drags on.
Fax	Fast reply assured. Message is clear, short. Shows agent is efficient. Reach daytime or at home.	Many authors may not have home fax. May intimidate if too strong. May sound like "get-rich" scheme.
E-mail	Fast reply assured. Impartial and businesslike. Reach worldwide clients. Easier for subsequent mail.	Many authors may not have e-mail. Detached and unfriendly. Viewed as unsolicited trash mail.
Phone call	Direct, warm, caring. Allow author catharsis. Sell services faster.	Therapist not literary agent. Hard to get commitment. Easy to feel author empathy and lower prices.

REFERENCES

Bankston, J. (1995). *Web browsing with Microsoft network.* New York: Prima Publishing.

Behram, A. (1995). *Web weavers: Creating dynamic web sites.* New York: New Riders Publishing.

Cool, L.C. (1986). *How to sell every magazine article you write.* Cincinnati, OH: Writer's Digest Books.

Cool, L.C. (1987). *How to write irresistible query letters.* Cincinnati, OH: Writer's Digest Books.

Cooper, J. (1996). Web power. *Cablevision, 20 (21),* 16-26.

Curtis, R. (1990). *Beyond the bestseller: A literary agent takes you inside the book business.* New York: NAL/Dutton.

Gray, D. (1996). *Web publishing with Adobe Pagemill.* Los Angeles, CA: Ventana Communications Group Inc.

Larsen, M. (1984). *How to be your own literary agent: The business of getting your book published.* New York: Houghton Mifflin Co.

Magid, J., Matthews, R.D., and Jones, P. (1995). *The web server book: Tools and techniques for building your own internet information site.* CA: Ventana Communications Group Inc.

Morris, M. (1996). *Web page design: A different multimedia.* NJ: Prentice-Hall.

Naujoks, A. and Ruben, D.H. (1996). *Hitler's Revenge.* Salt Lake City, UT: Northwest Publishing Incorporation.

Prevost, R. and McArdle, N.C. (1996). *The web design style guide: How to create a smash hit web site.* New York: McGraw-Hill.

Prima (development staff). (1996). *Web advertising and marketing.* New York: Prima Publishing.

Ruben, D.H. (1995). *Publicity for mental health clinicians: Using TV, radio, and print media to enhance your public image.* Binghamton, NY: The Haworth Press, Inc.

Ruben, D.H. and Reinbold, D. (1996). *One minute secrets to feeling great.* New York: Press-Tige Press.

Ruben, D.H. and Ruben, M.J. (1982). *Sixty Seconds to Success.* Westallis, WI: Pine Mountain Press.

Sosinsky, B. (1995). *Web browsing with America Online.* New York: Prima Publishing.

Stross, C. (1996). *The web architect handbook.* NJ: Addison-Wesley Publish ing.

Townsend, J. (1996). *Web site developers kit with Microsoft resources.* New York: SAMN.

Withers, J.P. (1995). *Web browsing with Prodigy: Exploring new worlds of graphics, text and sound on the World Wide Web.* New York: Prima Publishing.

PART II:
WRITING FOR MONEY

A year ago, I received a rejection from a publisher who said my manuscript was unsuitable for his press. "That's fine," I thought, "He's entitled to his own opinion." In fact, I hadn't given it much thought until I saw an attachment to the rejection letter. It was a copy of an article from a newspaper which the publisher had highlighted in yellow. So I read the particular passage with curiosity. My curiosity turned quickly to annoyance. There, in bold print, was written that reports of Jews dying in concentration camps (especially in gas chambers) were statistically inflated. The article went on to claim that 9 million, not 12 million, Jewish people perished at the hands of Nazi Germany.

Well, Holocaust statisticians may always bicker over numbers, and of course any historical tragedy sparks endless academic debate. But that's not what bothered me. Sure, it disturbed me whether the total death count was 9 million or 12 million. But what deeply disturbed me was *why that publisher sent me this newspaper reprint in the first place.*

Ask yourself this question: When you submit a manuscript to an impartial editor who doesn't know you from Adam, do you expect him or her to defensively correct your wrong ideas? No, of course not. Editors, publishers, and especially producers have so little time for replies that they are more cryptic. Letters state "Yes, let me see it," or "No, thank you."

But not everybody is like that. In academic publishing, you encounter the same problem. One editor sends a polite form letter rejecting the book and offers no reasons for its return. Another editor blasts you for audaciously for violating the sanctity of a theory or some diamond in the rough they have a claim on. Don't touch it, they exclaim, unless you are prepared to do it justice. Of course, what is justice to them may not be justice to somebody else.

That is why writing for money requires versatility. Sure, you need a market, but you also want a variety of options within that market from which you can decide for yourself which option is most suitable for your manuscript. The following chapters urge your instincts to go beyond having a good idea for a book, magazine article, software, video, or web property. Now is execution time. Construct your ideas in preliminary form, either in a proposal or e-mail inquiry letter, and be prepared to put it through the experimental test of your lifetime. Send it out for review.

If you're a veteran at scholarly or professional publishing, then you already have a sixth sense on what to expect. Naturally, editorial replies are less personable, less nurturing than many academic presses. This is because trade presses have 3,000 to 5,000 submissions compared to academic publishers receiving 300 to 1,000 submission per year. That does not mean your manuscript is a needle in a haystack. It would be, if you never had an insider's atlas on getting published.

Ahead in Chapters 4 through 8 you will hopefully find a treasure map leading you in the right direction to discover a wealthy pot of gold. The riches gained from any product you have published are derived, in part, from the pride in attaining your goal. But, frankly, pride is even better when you have cash to count. That's what earns the highest dividends on your investment in writing for money.

Chapter 4

Book Publishers

Today's emerging publishers are multimedia magnets. They attract a surge of energy from authors with traditional books, CDs, audio-tapes, software ideas, audio-visual programs, and scores of other configurations. This is what keeps their line of products one step above their high-tech competitors. Because publishing is survival of the fittest, some publishers ascend to comfortable plateaus, while others financially die. And, nothing stops the hunt for red-hot best-seller properties.

Editors are the biggest game hunters. They remain constantly on the lookout for prize-winning books. Sure, they may say their docket is full for two years. But face it; they're lying. They'd drop what they're doing if the authorized biography of President Clinton popped up. Who are they kidding?

With the world constantly in turmoil, news and advice keep us addicted to a steady diet of information coming from all forms of media. The media of books and especially self-help books command our attention in a different way: *We expect to be educated, entertained, and to feel better after reading a self-help book.* That's why buying consumers flock to discount booksellers such as Barnes & Noble and parade around the recovery sections. National surveys even propel this idea. One survey rated over 1,000 self-help books, sorting through the bewildering maze of titles (Santrock, Minnett, and Campbell, 1994). Results showed that buyers are picky about their selections and will return to that author or topic as long as they feel their needs are met.

Can you meet their needs? I believe you can. Whether your subject is step-parenting, self-esteem, or pregnancy, you can tap into the very soul of your reader and know what they really want. It begins with knowing precisely what books are successful and how your book can incorporate elements of their success into your own pages.

WHAT'S HOT, WHAT'S NOT

The *New York Times* bestseller list is an effective gauge of today's consumer taste buds. Appetites grow in leaps and bounds for certain self-help and how-to books, while other recovery titles peter out after months. But a short shelf life can be only a temporary setback. When the book's author or other health expert appears on TV reporting that some disorder is America's worst epidemic in centuries, watch what happens. It sets off a flurry of heal-seeking buyers for that not-so-good selling book. Now the book becomes a featured new release, even though it originally came out several months ago. What makes it popular today? Public awareness.

In this section, we discuss these red-hot books that the public wants. Admittedly, topics may not seem relevant to personal improvement or even reflect clinical trends in treatment. But so what? The sad truth is that these books *sell big, have sold big, and will continue to sell even bigger.* Let's consider what they are.

Love and Sex

Sexuality is king over buyer instincts. There's no question about it. Books sell big if they focus on lovemaking, infidelity, marriage, passion, lust, intimacy, dating, and pure, unadulterated sex from masturbation to eroticism. For example, sales of Dr. Keesling's *Sexual Pleasure* (1996) and *Sexual Healing* (1996) have hit mega-watts. Her other books boosted sales over 150,000 copies. Why, you ask? In part, it's the author. She's a sex therapist and previous surrogate partner for 12 years, has appeared on daytime talkies such as *Geraldo, Mike and Maty,* and was profiled in *Playboy* magazine. Add the sensual photographs included throughout her text and you have a near virtual-reality taste of love–just what Keesling and her publishers want you to get.

So why do Dr. Keesling's and other lovemaking series books stir excitement in readers? Is it because the subject matter is still taboo?

Not really. Sexual revolutions of the 1960s, 1970s, and 1980s broke the ice for the 1990s. Today, liberal sexual attitudes permit semipornography in self-improvement manuals. Generally, secular bookstores are very eager to shelve love and sexuality books and generously invite their authors for book signings. Even if books indirectly cover sex, themes of sex somehow emerge for publicity.

For instance, I recall a Barnes & Noble publicist arranging my book signing of *No More Guilt: Ten Steps to a Shame-Free Life.* Rather than publicize it as a "talk on guilt," we agreed that a larger audience would show up if the talk was on "how to rate your date." This was based on my last chapter. That publicist was right; people showed up.

Sexuality fits into almost every imaginable topic: relationships, religion, schools, home, the workplace, and illness. Capture intimate sensuality in your manuscript by devoting a section or entire chapter to the ecstasy, agony, and merry-go-round of emotions people suffer when sex and love mess up their lives.

Gay and Lesbian Lifestyles

In the last five years, marked by rising political gains by the gay rights movement, more publishers have come out of the closet with books on gays and lesbians. They are openly marketing fiction and nonfiction (recovery) books focused on lifestyles of homosexual partnerships. Lover relationship, secrecy versus lifting the iron curtain of shame, and the inner world of the dating scene are powerful reader selections. Buyers may or may not be homosexuals but they are definitely intrigued by this discriminated subculture and what lies ahead in their unending quest for public recognition.

Hate and Violence

Thank you, O.J. Simpson. There is no other way of saying it. Hate and violence topics were always somewhere on the shelf and represented a minority of autobiographic panoramas of abuse and dysfunction in celebrity families. But not until 1995's network airings of the O.J. Simpson trial and nightly commentaries by spindoctors did the American public wake up to the atrocities of domestic abuse.

Now the shelves are stuffed with books on parent abuse, child abuse, elderly abuse, divorce abuse, and any other emotionally debilitating effects abuse has on some population. In 1996, 29 books alone on violence were released, including books on violence and women, violence and gays, violence and disability, violence and religion, violence in the media, violence as obscenity, violence in schools, violence at work, violence in families, violence between intimates, violence prevention, and violence handbooks. Seasoned domestic abuse therapist Michael Paymar's *Violent No More* (1996) is one example. He advocates firm and swift rehabilitation for abusive men, while Tobias and Lalich's *Captive Hearts, Captive Minds* (1996) does the opposite. They take the victim's perspective, especially for cult survivors of abusive relationships.

The buzz words are that *untreated hate is a ticking time bomb for violence in a family.* Likewise, books on violence in the workplace are soaring. Murders and physical assaults at work have climbed to record highs, creating an urgent need for preventive action; one way is through handbooks. Teach employees safe practices to avert non-fatal or fatal assaults, especially individuals who handle money at their jobs. If you can plug these words or ideas into your manuscript, be prepared to receive many positive publisher replies.

Money and Power

Infomercial supercharger Anthony Robbins dominated the late-night airwaves with success-building gospel guaranteed to help buyers seek money and power: some did, some didn't, and some are still trying. But Tony Robbins is only one guru in the mind-power industry. His best-selling books typify the rise of greed-seeking harvesters who know there are two types of people in the world: winners and losers. Winners want books that push an upbeat attitude and that show insider secrets, tricks, and hands-on techniques for seizing happiness. Losers also are frantic buyers. They nosedive into power-surging books hoping to escape their misery, futility, and inferiority.

The power both types of consumers achieve or think they achieve is self-love. For them, it feels so intoxicating that they become addicted. They want more of the same. They run back to the bookstore for another dose of the author's medicine. Meaning and guidelines to power, wealth, and success must be in your book. Describe how these attributes are attainable. Describe what these things must feel like, and vicariously urge your reader to trust that, with courage and effort, they can live a caliber higher than ever imagined.

UFO and New Age

Thank you, *X-Files*. Fox TV's cult television hit show on the paranormal has renewed a generation of Roswell disbelievers into skywatching UFO experts. Agents Mulder and Scolly take us on a mystery tour filled with unexpected plot twists and encounters. We discover species far beyond the bizarre-o-sphere that 1960s audiences saw in *The Outer Limits* and *The Twilight Zone*. Now the tide has shifted. The government is involved; they are hiding things. And every episode of *X-Files* or its spinoff documentaries, such as film footage on alien autopsies, are nurturing the viewing public in the belief in UFOs and alien abduction.

Even Hollywood is picking up extraterrestrial vibes with recent releases of *Phenomenon* and *Independence Day*. Combine these with vintage science fiction films *2001: A Space Odyssey, Alien, Dr. Strangelove, Earth vs. The Flying Saucers, The Right Stuff!, The Day the Earth Stood Still, War of the Worlds, E.T.,* and *Close Encounters of the Third Kind*, and you'll see how disaster films of epic proportions have been a regular public obsession.

Whether it's 15-miles-in-diameter spaceships blotting out the skies or telepathic encounters with humanity, fascination abounds with alien invaders' superior technology. But the bottom line is this: tens of thousands of books sold in the last three years parallel the unquenchable thirst to know if life beyond our galaxies exist.

Commanding titles such as *The Andreasson Affair* (Fowler, 1994), *UFO Abductions in Gulf Breeze* (Walters and Walters, 1994), and *Alien Identities* (Thompson, 1994) send shivers up and down the spines of book browsers, tempting their insatiable curiosity. Feeding that curiosity are UFO gurus Whitley Streiber, Budd Hopkins, Dr. David Jacobs, and Dr. Raymond Fowler, among others. Each swears they are legitimately documenting investigations of people's abductions aboard UFOs. Are they? Are they really?

I know you're a skeptic. The peculiar part about UFO sightings for mental health experts is this: something is happening. A statistically significant number of patients previously living healthy lives are now suffering trauma. They are not war veterans. They have not been in car accidents or been raped or suffered post-traumatic conditions normally diagnosed. No, they claim something else.

They claim to be victims of alien abduction, and they *aren't kidding either.* These are not delusional, psychotic people. They are mothers, fathers, and are employed in normal jobs. They are functionally adaptive except that they have unusually bizarre flashbacks and nightmares about being strapped down on a surgical table and having needles stuck into them. And that's only the beginning. Some even claim the surgeons were either "grays" (referring to gray, little aliens) or reptile-looking aliens. Okay Scottie, beam me back to reality. I've had enough! Maybe it's enough. But it makes you think, doesn't it?

The point is this: While intuitively you may want to dismiss this mumbo jumbo and insist that these people "get a life," remember who these people are. They own a big share of the book buyers' market. These unrelenting believers head straight for the new-age shelf and can't wait for updates on UFO sightings, abduction experiences, and crop circles. Whether you personally or clinically agree or disagree with their stories, be open-minded enough to explore their insights. Devote a chapter or book to the weird symptoms of their sudden, abnormally shifting lifestyles.

The Devil, God, and the Spiritual World

Another thriving twist of new-age literature is devil worship. Readers fascinated with satanism from the standpoint of participant and the religiously exonerated are tripling book sales in religious gift shops. Exorcism, in particular, seems to be a raging craze. Southern readers top the list. Fundamental Baptists recently have been upset by fears of satanic uprising, witnessed, they believe, by out-of-control teen homicides, church burnings, adolescent pregnancies, and devil worshipers performing barbaric rituals. Reflecting these concerns are spiritually based books guiding parents, teens, clergy, and all civilized men to take precautions against widespread demonic destruction.

Since demonism draws a strong readership, mostly in the Bible-belt states, consider covering satanic activities in your book. In parenting books, for example, feature interviews with former satanic members whose retrospection may be helpful to parents of today's teens. Or, if writing on anger and aggression, explore the intimidating threats and acts of murder, rape, and cemetery desecrations frequently done by devil worshippers. Knowing that your topic revolves in some way around antidemonic messages can broaden your target audience.

The Three V's: Victim, Vulnerable, and Vindication

Books on death, dying, and bereavement have a long history of popularity. They heal the ailing heart of a person suffering recent losses or facing the painfully slow deterioration of friends or relatives with cancer. Books on death and dying also speak to a common thread that is now addressed in fast-selling recovery books. This thread is the three V's: victim, vulnerable, and vindication. All three topics must converge for the book's impact to be effective.

Think of it this way: The first part of the book describes how inescapable trauma tragically afflicts a person or group of people. The middle section elaborates on their downward emotional spiral, in which they lose jobs, self-respect, or go through a series of failures. Now the best part: In remaining chapters, you show how underdogs resurrect their strength using hands-on strategies. They can *and will* rise above the odds of self-doubt to a vindicated new self who is better than before. Sound like a fiction book? Not really. Try true stories. Consider the many children who were autistic and are now functional, or closed-head-injured victims who under vigilant care make a swift recuperation. Of course, damaging paralysis will never be hopeless again now that patients are inspired by spinal-chord-injured celebrity Christopher Reeves. All of these reborn winners followed the path of being a victim, vulnerable, and are boldly vindicated.

True Crime

As crime spreads its ugly trail from urban to rural localities, readers have developed a morbid fascination for details of carnage. Books about serial killers, rapists, pedophiles, and even gang killings rank higher with those who love to read about violent crime than books about Mafioso (Bintliff, 1993; Wilson, 1992). Ten to 15 years ago, mob hits were the talk of literary tables, lead by trail-blazing works such as *The Godfather*. Since the arrest of New York Mafia head John Gotti, few remarkable stories of mobs have hit the press. Instead, sensationalism has shifted to inhumane crimes of decapitation, cannibalism, and senseless drive-by shootings motivated by drug money.

In all crime-based writing, there is a basic formula tying human motive with social reaction (Corvasce and Paglino, 1995; Wingate, 1992). It is the same formula used by corrections officers in memorizing the penal code for different degrees of crime, that is, PKRN. PKRN stands for the following:

1. Purposely = suspects acted with premeditation.
2. Knowingly = suspects may or may not have committed the action but were aware of the crime in progress.
3. Recklessly = suspects deliberately were abusive of something.
4. Negligently = intentional or not, suspect overlooked something critical leading to a problem.

PKRN is an excellent guide in analytically probing the personality of criminals and arriving at conclusions that can help stop potential crime suspects. Sure, you can expand on these variables for a crime-reading public, but take it one step farther. While it is entertaining for some, let it be a self-help survival guide for high-risk teens, young adults, and even repeat offenders aching for solid, how-to directions.

CADILLAC VS. CHEVY PUBLISHERS

Debate always rages about where to place your manuscript. One camp swears that the only fruitful publishing house is a large-scale, Manhattan-based publisher. They are equipped with all the bells and whistles for production and publicity. Other writing aficionados praise small presses for their individual attention paid to first-time authors and bend-over-backwards efforts to visibly market a book.

Opinions remain split largely for two reasons. First is that authors believe a full-service publishing house such as Macmillan, Random

House, Doubleday, HarperCollins, and Simon & Schuster have cornered the marketplace and can muscle in on wholesalers and distributors, given their reputation and track record. Their high volume sales command powerful respect among book promoters.

While undoubtedly there is merit to this opinion, ask yourself if larger is really better. The Cadillac companies create a curriculum of sorts through which authors diligently follow step-by-step in sequence, with each phase of preproduction or production involving separate editors. By the time the book cover is ready, editors from publicity already have mapped out a media package hopefully tuned to reach your market. Author input is welcome, but editors in each division already follow a fairly definitive regimen based on previous marketing and may seem arrogantly robotic about their plans.

Authors who enjoy being led like sheep by a trusting shepherd have nothing to fear. They just follow the row of arrows painted on the floor around the confusing maze until door number one or door number two is opened for them. Rational thinking is an accessory. You don't really need it. You have already put months of mental sweat and tears into writing this book and now you can just sit back and enjoy the cruise.

The only other disadvantage besides not having an active voice in production is that you relinquish not only the copyright but also your control over book circulation. By contrast, control is with you all the time using smaller publishers. They actively recruit, depend on, and expect your principal decision making in every stage of book processing.

The second reason for using small presses is this: Smaller presses such as Adams Publishing, Contemporary Books, Dartnell Corporation, Health Communications, and Human Services Institute limit their targeted buyers. They narrow in on, for example, health care professionals or some career or demographic sample rather than globally distributing books over the entire reading continent.

That's true; they do that and they do it well. There are legitimate reasons why small publishers do this. Take, for example, Florida-based magazine and publishing pathfinder Health Communications. They've enjoyed rising profits and crank out 30 to 40 book titles a year. They have capitalized on a prime buying market. Thousands of recovering alcoholics, families in transition, and heartbroken, therapy-seeking codependents rely on Health Communications' how-to books. Books advise readers on rapid ways to change their lives. Advice appears from renowned professionals and celebrities who currently have either monthly columns or guest articles in the publisher's several trade and lay magazines. Smart editors know that if you continue to familiarize loyal magazine subscribers with certain people's names and those names are also book authors, book sales will skyrocket.

The Haworth Press, publisher of this book, does the same thing. They've gained prestige in academic and trade quadrants through their "journal factory." They produce new journals, keeping up with current trends in business, mental health, and allied fields. Original peer-reviewed articles are frequently authored by the same individuals whose books are deliberately advertised at the front, middle, or back of the journal. They also know what they're doing and have remained a pillar of strength in the small press industry. No, they don't have unlimited funds for a supernova media campaign, booking you on flights and national talk shows. That's not their style. But they don't need to do that, for the following reason.

If your paperback trade has *Publisher's Weekly* quoting its high sales and it enters a second production run of say 3,000 to 10,000 copies, small press publishers know that word of this success will spread like wildfire. The first to hear of this are the American Booksellers Association (ABA) and reprint publishers (McCollister, 1995).

ABA is always on the lookout for prolific books since literary and theatrical agents are breathing down its neck for properties. Agents want properties adaptable for TV, video, or motion picture. That's how novelist-screenwriter David Klass, whose novels include *Samurai Inc.* and *The Atami Dragons,* signed a two-picture screenwriting deal with Universal Studios for six figures. Or why Patrick Johnson's half-written Navy novel *The Nimitz Class* was optioned by Universal for $250,000 against $500,000, plus a $250,000 bonus on the first day before the cameras.

That is only one way nonfiction properties catapult from small press stardom. Reprint publishers also get into the act. Companies such as Bantam and Vintage, among others, literally purchase the copyright on a book, which they in turn reprint under their banner in mass quantities (20,000 to 100,000 copies, if not more per run).

Copyright purchases all vary, but the standard deal is an outright cash settlement between small press and reprint publisher, where you, the author, and your publisher split the proceeds 50/50. That means if annual royalty checks paid you a respectable $1,000 to $3,000 purely on sales generated by your publisher, and now a reprint company buys it lock, stock, and barrel for $250,000, guess what that means? You instantly win the jackpot of $125,000. And it's still not over. Clever negotiations usually reserve dribbling royalty earnings to both small press publisher and author on all future reprint sales. So, besides your windfall, you now can plan on a limited-life, annual check from the reprint publisher based on net or gross book sales.

Does it really matter if you choose a Chevy or a Cadillac as long as the dollars pay off? I don't think it does. Personally, I have found working intimately with small and medium-sized presses extremely rewarding, profitable, and easier to work with. In starting from scratch, smaller companies have real-live voices at the other end of the telephone receiver with whom you can discuss your proposal, even if they reject it on the spot. Don't delude yourself into thinking that name-brand publishers are the only trampoline to jump-start your writing career. Yes, they can do it. Yes, they are glamorous. And yes, you will taste a bit of glitzy Hollywood life and be treated like royalty. But once the glitter fades and you return to bottom-line profits, enterprising small presses with a niche market may put more than change in your pocket.

GHOSTWRITING AND EDITING

In the last chapter, we discussed the many advantages of being an editor and ghostwriter, including creative marketing avenues to stimulate client referrals. With your juices stirring, consider the actual nuts and bolts of the job from proposal to contract and many common roadblocks authors throw in your path along the way. The good news is that solutions exist for these roadblocks. The bad news is that you can't avoid them.

Ghostwriting Outline and Contract

Congratulations. You've made an award-winning pitch to a failing author who is convinced you can raise the sun, reach the stars, and fulfill his publishing dreams. And, quite frankly, you feel absolutely certain you can do it. Now comes the "put your money where your mouth is" part of listing step by step what you plan to perform for the author (see Figure 4.1).

Ghostwriting proposals contain two sections and are prepared and mailed to authors prior to issuing a contract. The first section sequentially describes the order that the author can expect after you begin the project. This includes (but is not limited to) method of delivery for ideas or draft manuscripts (diskette, hard-copy, other), whether person-to person contact is necessary, your role as either ghostwriter or second author, and role as literary agent or marketer after the manuscript is approved.

The second section lists all substantial costs incurred at each phase of the project. Fees are usually not estimates but may be negotiable, depending on the authors' special needs. Authors may hire you at the outset to establish a marketing and media tour plan or to prepare submission packages for simultaneous publisher submissions.

Independent Contract Agreement

Upon receipt of the author's approval of the proposal, send a standard contract similar to that in Figure 4.2. As with all legal documents, be sure your version undergoes scrutiny by a trusted attorney, preferably one specializing in publishing or entertainment law.

The contract opens by defining the parties in the agreement and proceeds through a series of clauses and subclauses clearly explaining the responsibilities of ghostwriter and author. It includes the compensation schedule at each phase of manuscript completion. Note the critical indemnification clause (1.1.7.). Here the author understands he will hold the independent contractor (ghostwriter) harmless in the event any claims are brought against the work. Commonly, this clause protects the ghostwriter from unforeseen

FIGURE 4.1. Proposal to rewrite manuscript

BEST IMPRESSIONS INTERNATIONAL INCORPORATED

4211 OKEMOS ROAD, SUITE 22, OKEMOS, MICHIGAN 48864, U.S.A.
PHONE or FAX: 517-347-0944; PHONE: 1-800-595-BEST

Book/Rewrite Proposal
for
The Female Trap

Steps of Book

1. Hire myself, scriptdoctor at Best Impressions International Inc. as ghostwriter or co-writer so that story line falls into place and flows for immediate placement with publisher. Scripting is done by you sending the manuscript either on diskette (preferable) or as typewritten text. On many occasions, as when I start from scratch with authors, frequently we meet at your home for consultation.

2. After the story is edited, revised on contract, and drafts approved, our firm locates a publisher or multimedia outlet. We work with two types of publishers: standard royalty and coventure. Standard royalty publishers pay very little and rarely accept first time authors unless the book contains a powerful angle. Coventure publishers pay 70% and authors pay 30% of production costs. This arrangement allows the author more control, as well as the ability to recover costs and money faster and more reliably.

   In the event that we wish to skip a publisher and seek a TV producer, arrangements are made to adapt your book into a screenplay or teleplay.

3. When manuscript is accepted and published, we either work with publisher in marketing or offer to you a personalized marketing service. We also make contacts through our multimedia networks.

Costs of Book

1. Submission to publisher (traditional or subsidy) and negotiation/ consultation with acquisitions editor is free.

FIGURE 4.1 (continued)

2. Standard editorial and ghostwriting services are as follows:

    a. Upon signing contract, **$2,000**
    b. Upon approval of first draft, **$500**
    c. Upon approval of final draft, **$500**
    d. If manuscript not on diskette, optiscan cost is $1.75/page.
    e. Best Impressions retains 10% on domestic and 20% subsidiary right on royalty earnings on books. Adaptations as play or screenplay treated under separate contract.
    f. Travel and lodging for visit with author at author's expense

3. Marketing options and prices are available upon request.

4. Conversion of manuscript into play or screenplay (teleplay), **$1,000**.

All terms are spelled out clearly in our standard contract, sent upon your approval of this proposal.

FIGURE 4.2. Sample contract for independent contractor agreement

BEST IMPRESSIONS INTERNATIONAL INCORPORATED

4211 OKEMOS ROAD, SUITE 22, OKEMOS, MICHIGAN 48864, U.S.A.
PHONE or FAX: 517-347-0944; PHONE: 1-800-595-BEST

Independent Contractor Agreement

AGREEMENT IS MADE this sixth day of June, 1996. The following outlines this agreement:

1.0 The INDEPENDENT CONTRACTOR has been retained by Mr. X (AUTHOR), as an independent contractor for the project of write, edit, and find publisher for the manuscript tentatively titled *Stocks, Bonds, and Jail* (subsequently referred to as the "work").

1.1 The contractor will be responsible for successfully completing said project according to specifications. Specifications, approval steps, and reimbursement schedule read as follows:

    1.1.1. GENERAL OUTLINE AND DIRECTION: Scripted out is proposed direction of work, proposed synopsis of work, and general outline of work, featuring basic elements of the work designed for mass media audience.

Upon Approval: $2,000.00. *Timetable: Due upon signing of contract*

    1.1.2. DETAILED OUTLINE: Specific and categorically complete chapter descriptions with design, graphics (if necessary), how-to methods, scripted out for review and approval.

Upon Approval: $500. *Timetable: 1 to 2 weeks*

    1.1.3. FIRST DRAFT: Preedited version of document containing exact chapter narrative, format, examples of methods used, and placement of graphics (if any) following the detailed outline. First-draft corrections are covered by this section. Request for **second** and **subsequent** drafts cost **$250** per draft revision.

Upon Approval: $1,500 (for completion of first draft). *Timetable: 6 to 8 weeks*

FIGURE 4.2 (continued)

1.1.4. FINAL DRAFT/PUBLISHER CONTACT: Editorial changes incorporated into chapter text with corrections received from AUTHOR. Camera-ready manuscript delivered on diskette using Macintosh (Microsoft Word 5.0) or hard copy prepared according to publisher specifications for layout. There are three steps involved in seeking publisher. First, publisher prospectus and cover letter is designed ($300). Second, an agency retainer fee is obtained ($25) for seeking publisher. Third, contact is made with standard royalty and coventure publishers.

Upon Approval $1,000 (Final draft). *Timetable: 3 weeks*

Inquiry/prospectus materials	**$300**
Agency Retainer Fee	**$25**
	$1,325

1.1.5. REVISIONS REQUESTED BY PUBLISHER: Editorial changes will be requested by publisher to prepare for camera-ready submission. Amounts will be determined after publishing contract is signed. Author is not responsible for paying these amounts before the contract. Terms will be outlined in a separate addendum.

Upon Approval: To be determined (in separate addendum to contract)

1.1.6. TRAVEL, LODGING, MEALS: Round-trip visit to author/publisher's location or research location for consultation on manuscript. Round trip plus expenses (lodging, meals) to be paid for by author. Round-trip travel is from Lansing to wherever research is based (if necessary). Arrangements can be made by AUTHOR or by INDEPENDENT CONTRACTOR. All costs paid in advance by AUTHOR by credit card or cashier's check.

Approved Flight Cost: to be determined. *Timetable: Determined upon signing contract and arrangements made with INDEPENDENT CONTRACTOR*

Lodging/Meals: paid by author.

1.1.6.1. All subsequent trips requested by the author for consultation or book promotion outside of 100-mile radius of Lansing to follow similar reimbursement schedule whereby INDEPENDENT CONTRACTOR promises to find lowest cost flight (or equivalent transportation), lodging, and meals upon approval of AUTHOR. (NOTE: Publishers usually pay this fee.)

1.1.7. AUTHOR indemnifies the INDEPENDENT CONTRACTOR, and agrees to hold the INDEPENDENT CONTRACTOR harmless in the event that any claims are brought against the work.

1.2 Other terms agreed upon include the following:

1.2.1. INDEPENDENT CONTRACTOR is a co-author of book and will have his or her name appear as second author on cover of book and on title page.

1.2.2. INDEPENDENT CONTRACTOR receives 30% (15% as agent, 15% as ghostwriter) of publisher advances offered to AUTHOR. INDEPENDENT CONTRACTOR receives 30% of author's royalty of gross book sales except returns (e.g., if author receives 10% royalty from publisher, INDEPENDENT CONTRACTOR receives 3%, and AUTHOR receives 7%).

1.2.3. INDEPENDENT CONTRACTOR reserves the right of first refusal to write, assist, or consult on any screenplay or other audiovisual property (e.g., software, CD, audioscript, radio show) derived or adapted from the work. Terms of royalty split on derivative works or subsidiary rights is 50/50, including but not limited to paperback reproductions, foreign rights sales, serializations, teleplay and screenplay options, outright purchases, or other multimedia adaptations and representations.

1.2.4. INDEPENDENT CONTRACTOR to receive 10 complimentary copies of the work upon its publication.

1.2.5. INDEPENDENT CONTRACTOR to procure offers from either traditional royalty publishers or coventure publishers for AUTHOR to approve. Final decision with publisher rests with AUTHOR. INDEPENDENT CONTRACTOR to attempt contacts with producers or through his or her contacts procure interest in teleplay or screenplay adaptation.

1.2.6. INDEPENDENT CONTRACTOR reserves right of first refusal to give a price quote on personal marketing of the work through

FIGURE 4.2 (continued)

Best Impressions International Inc.'s Media Services Division. Prices for contact with radio, TV, or other media agreed upon with author will appear as an addendum to this contract.

AUTHOR will not deduct or withhold any taxes, FICA, or other deductions. INDEPENDENT CONTRACTOR will not be entitled to any fringe benefits, such as unemployment insurance, medical insurance, pension plans, or other such benefits offered under employment situation.

During this project, INDEPENDENT CONTRACTOR may be in contact with or directly working with proprietary information that is important to this work and competitive works by other publishers. All information will be treated with strict confidence and may not be used at any time or in any manner in work INDEPENDENT CONTRACTOR may do with others in the industry.

Agreed:

_____   Date: June 6, 1996
Douglas H. Ruben, PhD
Independent Contractor

_____   Date: June 6, 1996
Mr. X

_____
Social Security Number

low royalty sales, publisher problems, or negative media reactions lambasting the book or author.

In "Other terms agreed upon," note the specification of what role the independent contractor will serve, in this case as second author. Besides fee for service, royalty earnings are made clear both as ghostwriter (co-author) and in serving as literary agent. Another clause conveniently reserves your right to refuse or accept helping the author market his or her book, even if the publisher has a publicity division. Finally, when all is said and done, remember that terms spelled out here define an independent contract relationship, not an employer/employee relationship with the author. The author does not make any withholdings of compensation nor dictate the hours, location, or tasks governing the ghostwriter's job.

Contracts vary by the focus of your work. Where the focus is on literary agent, plus any additional services provided, such as submission packages and editing, spell out exactly what the agent does (see Figure 4.3). Identify, for example, terms of hiring, types of materials author can expect agent to prepare, use of language such as "net profits," and length of agreement. Clearly defining your job duties and compensation, as always, eliminates needless ambiguity at the outset before the project launches into action.

Roadblocks to Author Happiness

Contracts begin, but do not guarantee, a smooth-sailing process. After a signed agreement is returned, along with your first cash installment, you'd think you were ready to begin. But suddenly the telephone rings: "Incidentally, I forgot to mention this earlier, but can you . . . ?" You patiently listen, troubleshoot in your mind the most professional but least costly solution on your part, and realize that months of eleventh-hour questions and roadblocks are inevitable. Below are the most common roadblocks arising during all phases of a ghostwriting or editorial contract. Let's see what they are and how to respond to them.

1. "It doesn't look the same as when I gave it to you."
2. "I want another rewrite."
3. "Can you do research? . . . I don't think I have enough."

4. "I don't have a word processor, just hard copy pages."
5. "I want this type of publisher only."
6. "I'll pay you later, can you keep working on the project?"
7. "Can you travel here to get materials or talk with me?"
8. "Will you be the spokesperson for this book?"

"It Doesn't Look the Same as When I Gave It to You."

Manuscripts are precious jewels. Parchment to you, perhaps, but to authors who slaved over an idea or manuscript for months and years, it holds powerful sentimental value. They've created it, nurtured it, even fantasized about it. They picture it wrapped beautifully in a dust jacket with their name across the binding. Parental love, affection, and sacrifice all describe their emotional bond toward this child. Now, with anxiety, they've agreed to part from their cherished offspring. In your hands, in your judgment, they entrust you with their diamond where before nobody has had this privilege.

Think this is a little much? Well, it's probably not enough. Words alone cannot adequately describe the passion authors feel toward a manuscript and why they are so disturbed when you make changes. At the outset, it is recommended that you clearly state in conversation and even on the proposal that manuscript revisions may look very different from the author's original copy. Remind authors of this transformation so that when they receive your first draft, they won't gasp, "My God! What happened?"

"I Want Another Rewrite"

On original works dictated by the author—that is, where there were no original manuscripts to work from—ghostwriters have to be engineers as well as writers. They calculate ideas in an orderly outline, plotting out sections of the book, which develop plot, characters, and follow any important events chronologically. Organization of note taking and reframing the notes in a literary portrait attempts to match the mental story line already in the author's mind. When your composition disagrees with the author's mental story line or details are out of place, naturally you must correct these mistakes for accuracy.

FIGURE 4.3. Sample contract to use for independent agency and service agreement

BEST IMPRESSIONS INTERNATIONAL INCORPORATED

4211 OKEMOS ROAD, SUITE 22, OKEMOS, MICHIGAN 48864, U.S.A.
PHONE or FAX: 517-347-0944; PHONE: 1-800-595-BEST;
E-MAIL: mjruben@aol.com

Independent Agency and Service Contract

THIS AGREEMENT is made this 18th day of July, 1996 by and between Dr. X, residing at X address (herein called AUTHOR) and Douglas H. Ruben, residing at Best Impressions International Inc., 4211 Okemos Road, Suite 22, City of Okemos, State of Michigan 48864 (herein called AGENT).

WITNESSETH

NOW THEREFORE, in consideration of the promises, and of the mutual undertakings herein contained, and for other good and valuable considerations, the parties agree as follows:

1.0 *Terms of hiring:* AGENT will endeavor to seek a bona fide and appropriate offer of employment in any field or fields in which the AGENT is authorized to represent the AUTHOR. Employment involves placement of manuscript with publisher, producer, or acting in writing, consulting capacity for multiple jobs. The type of writings usually done by AUTHOR, prestige of program, publisher, or motion picture involved, AUTHOR's professional standing in the field and AUTHOR's customary salary or compensation will all be weighed in the entertainment industry market schedule of minimums. AGENT agrees to submit to AUTHOR any offers received. No agreement shall bind AUTHOR without the AUTHOR's written consent and signature.

1.0.1. AUTHOR should be ready, able, and willing and available to render his or her services. His or her refusal or inability to present himself or herself for interviews, possible layoffs due to strikes, or leaves of absence is the responsibility of the AUTHOR.

1.0.2. AGENT shall not require an AUTHOR to execute a release with respect to any literary material owned by the AUTHOR, submitted by such AUTHOR to the AGENT. Nothing herein shall be deemed to prevent an AGENT from submitting to the AUTHOR release forms required by a third party.

1.0.3. AGENT shall not communicate to others information relating to the affairs of the AUTHOR, which the AUTHOR has requested the AGENT not to communicate to others. However, the foregoing shall not prohibit the AGENT from divulging any information in arbitration or before a government body or official or accredited representative of a government body or official.

FIGURE 4.3 (continued)

(2) Independent Agency Agreement

1.0.4. AGENT shall act with reasonable diligence, care, and skill at all times in the interest of his or her AUTHOR and shall not act against the AUTHOR's interests. He or she shall consult with the AUTHOR at reasonable times and intervals during normal business hours and shall advance and protect the interest to the said AUTHOR in the radio, television, publisher, or motion picture fields in which he or she is authorized to represent said limits of his authority and shall keep AUTHOR informed of the progress made on his or her behalf.

1.0.5. At the written request of the AUTHOR, the AGENT shall give the AUTHOR, in writing, information stating what efforts the AGENT has made on behalf of the AUTHOR within a reasonable time preceding such request, and the AGENT shall inform the AUTHOR of the status of all negotiations made on behalf of the AUTHOR during such period and reasonable details as to the terms of the deals being negotiated, if any. Such information shall include the names of the persons spoken with by the AGENT on behalf of the AUTHOR with an approximate date for such conversations.

1.1 **Materials prepared:** AGENT will prepare preliminary synopses or other promotional materials sufficient for submission to publishers, producers, production companies, or other parties assigned by AGENT through whom the book, screenplay/teleplay contract may be procured. AUTHOR will supply AGENT a copy of the full manuscript and other such materials requested to aid in proper exposure of said work.

1.1.1 Submission Package and Manuscript Editing: AGENT will prepare a submission package according to specifications supplied by AUTHOR, using questionnaire, personal interview, or other tools requested by AGENT. AGENT also will edit three chapters provided by AUTHOR.

1.2 **Commissions and Compensation:** Payment of $100.00 will be paid to AGENT upon execution of contract to defray clerical costs incurred in promotion of publisher, screenplay/teleplay proposal. Other commissions include:

1.2.1.a. Commission may be paid on moneys received by the AUTHOR or publication/production deals that have been negotiated by the AGENT.

1.2.1.b. May be paid for purchase of script, book manuscript, either a one-time buy or over-scale options, net profit, residuals, and royalties payments.

1.2.1.c. In all cases, commissions will be 15% (fifteen percent) of AUTHOR's total compensation, which the AGENT has negotiated. Payments directed to AGENT will be sent to AUTHOR. Where possible, split checks will be sent to AGENT and AUTHOR.

Other compensations include:

1.2.2. Fee for submission package is $200; fee for chapter editing is $50 per chapter. Fee for three edited chapters is $150. Additional chapters not

(3) Independent Agency Agreement

exceeding 25 double-spaced pages is $50; chapters exceeding 25 double-spaced pages is $60 per chapter. Fees for chapters in excess of 75 pages or involving technical information are negotiable.

1.2.2.a. Edited version of document reflects spelling, grammar, and other stylistic changes tailored for publisher submission. Style guidelines conform with the genre of book (fiction, nonfiction, etc.) and type of publisher selected (trade, academic, etc.). Author will receive galley proofs for correction of technical and basic story line information. Request for **second** and **subsequent** rewritten drafts cost **$250** per draft revision.

1.3. For purposes of this agreement: "Net profits" shall be computed, determined, and paid in accordance with definition of net profits defined in the production/distribution agreement between production company and the distributor or buyer of the picture, provided that these terms equal or exceed WGA guidelines for writer's contracts. Additional payments for sequels, remakes, pilots, series, and other television or motion picture uses of the work are subject to terms defined in subsequent production/distribution agreements.

1.4 Length of the agreement: AUTHOR to entitle AGENT to full and exclusive rights for procuring a publisher/producer for a period of six months beginning the date of execution of this agreement. After which, renewal of this contract is contingent upon approval of both parties either by addendum or issuance of a new contract.

1.5 Indemnification and dispute: AUTHOR indemnifies and holds harmless AGENT in the event that any claims are brought against the work or process of finding a producer. Any controversy or claim arising out of or relating to this agreement or any breach thereof shall be settled by arbitration in accordance with the rules of the American Arbitration Association, and judgment upon the award rendered by the arbitrators may be entered in any court having jurisdiction thereof. The prevailing party shall be entitled to reimbursement of costs and reasonable attorneys' fees.

1.6 Binding: This agreement shall inure to the benefit of, and shall be binding upon, the executors, survivors, administrators, and assigns of the parties.

1.7 Nonpartnership: Nothing herein contained shall be construed to create a partnership between the parties. Their relation shall be one independent contracting of services. AUTHOR will not deduct or withhold any taxes, FICA, or other deductions. As an independent contractor, you will not be entitled to any fringe benefits such as unemployment insurance, medical insurance, pension plans, or other such benefits that would be offered under employment situation.

FIGURE 4.3 (continued)

(3) Independent Agency Agreement

1.8   *Total Agreement:* This agreement constitutes the entire understanding of the parties.

In WITNESS WHEREOF, the parties hereunto set their respective hand and seal this 18th day of July, 1996.

_____
Douglas H. Ruben, PhD
AGENT
366 48 0962

_____
Dr. X
AUTHOR

_____
Social Security Number

However, corrections for omission of fact or faults in story line are not usually a sore area. Ghostwriters just make the changes and think nothing of it. Problems arise when, overall, authors believe the draft "just doesn't sound right." Compared to what? Compared to their inner voice saying "I want it different." Are you obliged to follow their wishes and redraft a new chapter or book until their palates are content? Yes and no. Yes, you are under contract to procure a finished version or else they do not have to pay you; but, "no," frequent rewrites beyond corrections of fact or story line are not gratis. Built into the contract is a clause (see Figure 4.2, clause 1.1.3) explicitly stating that requests for "second and subsequent drafts cost $250 per draft revision."

It's a penalty against the author for being picky. Penalties are meant to discourage repetitive and needless requests for rewrites. Another reason authors want rewrites is because they object to your writing style or believe you are depicting their characters or themselves (biography) incorrectly. However, hopefully they had time to preview your other written work before signing your contract. If not, explain that a particular style you may have coalesces with what publishers want and already exists in the marketplace.

As for depiction of characters, ghostwriters need creative freedom in cleaning up one-dimensional, static, and boring characters. They frequently stretch their literary license to imaginative limits. Authors may not know this ahead of time and could benefit from understanding the ghostwriter's objective.

"Can You Do Research? . . . I Don't Think I Have Enough"

Nonfiction books strongly grounded in research must represent the facts correctly and cite references where the facts are drawn from. For example, on *Hunger: The Paradox of Plenty* (White-Stevens, 1996), I served as ghostwriter and editor on a *festschrift* for a particular scholar.

Each chapter was a commentary on the state of agricultural science, derived from theoretical and applied research. When the text directly corresponded to the references, words flowed smoothly and intelligibly. But chapter authors also made quantum leaps in commentaries that were irrelevant to the citations. Knowing next to nothing about agriculture, I had to ask the author who hired me for more data. There had to be some way I could document their critical thinking to primary or secondary sources. She provided them; but, were she to request I find them, research service would add on to the cost.

"I Don't Have a Word Processor, Just Hard-Copy Pages"

Today's generation of authors are sophisticated computer users who know how to operate word processing software or e-mail on servers. They will gladly ship you notes, figures, or even a working manuscript on diskette for your editorial convenience. No big deal, and that represents half the authors.

Now for the remainder–"computerphobics," I call them. They toyed with the notion of learning artificial intelligence back in the days of IBM punch cards (1960s, mid 1970s) but didn't like it. Frankly, I don't blame them. They were already masters of the typewriter and were eagerly pleased with the invention of self-correcting, electric typewriters, so now their labor was cut down enormously, and that's where they fixated at.

Authors who regretfully are apologetic about not using computers or having their manuscript on diskette (typed, say, by somebody else), run into a problem. Sure, you can generously offer to retype their manuscript from scratch. If you're writing a brand new story using their manuscript as a guideline, that is not a bad idea. In editing jobs, this can't be done without wasted, unpaid time.

Two solutions are at your fingertips. First is to charge the author $2.50 to $3.00 per page for typing it. Second is to optiscan it using any number of full-page scanners at a cost of $1.75 to $2.00 per page (see Figure 4.1, section 2d under "Costs of Book"). Presuming you have a scanner, the speed of feeding the sheets through one at a time or in groups should be equal to a reasonable fee for service. Without a scanner in your computer arsenal, costs for renting equipment become outrageous, and the author is better advised to have you type the pages.

"I Want This Type of Publisher Only"

Inexperienced authors may insist on finding a large-scale, Cadillac publisher. They reason that a dust-cover, hardback book with their glossy black-and-white picture on the back instantly commands multifigure sales. When you explain that small presses offer personalized attention, whereas larger firms give a number and ask you to stand in line, authors may accept the rationality and concede. But when logical explanation repeatedly is futile, simply agree to submit inquiries to both small timers and Manhattan's finest. You already know who will respond and the formal rejection letters act as proof-positive of your intuition.

"I'll Pay You Later, Can You Keep Working on the Project?"

There is an unwritten rule regulating freelance work: *Never do work on spec.* Speculative work is where payment for service is deferred until a later time. In the real world, this happens for two reasons. The first is that an author's current finances are unexpectedly low and projected to improve in a month or so. Wholesome promises of later payment give authors time to borrow, steal, or somehow cough up dollars owed to you. But how do you know they will do that? What if authors lose their jobs, go bankrupt, become physically disabled, or suffer other personal disasters? Calamities of life may build reassuring mountains of payment delays in the form of contract addenda and IOUs, but this paperwork is essentially worthless.

Sooner or later you'll want your reimbursement. Do you sue the delinquent client? No. Courts may rule your contract is binding and order payment be made, but how do you squeeze blood from a turnip? It means taking a loss after spending hours of time, energy, and money on a wasted project.

A second reason for deferment is overzealous projections of the book's sales record. Clients excited about their concept get evangelical. They are defensively positive their book will be a blockbuster bestseller, earning millions of dollars. Recently, for example, I heard from a matchmaker mogul out west insisting that her how-to secrets on long-lasting dating would be a bestseller. She would only work with co-writers willing to "go the distance and take the risk." In other words, she refused to pay me a dime.

This propaganda has deep fish hooks for new ghostwriters and is the work of a speculative shark. Such speculative predators lure eager writers into their feeding nest and slowly nibble away at your patience. They ravage in many types, the following among them:

a. *The lachrymal lamprey:* This eely character has sharp teeth and ready tears. He or she woos you, almost on a daily basis. Not a day goes by without a call from this person who beats you down until you agree to the suggestion that you write a complete submission package or even a first chapter. Once you do, that will determine if the lamprey likes you. If not, well, hey, you can afford to pay for your own creative time, can't you?

b. *The loudmouthed louse:* This person is a vicarious entrepreneur. Without investing a dime personally, this person has put together several authors under his or her empire. All that's needed is your creative genius for another piece of the larger puzzle or to get things rolling. Shrewdly, you refuse to do spec work. But after hearing how this louse is already half way to the publishing goal, you decide the job is not time-consuming and agree to be a patsy. Sooner than later, you see that this person has other freelancers duplicating your work, all on the free-salary system. Aggravating, to say the least.

Avoid speculative parasites by always asking for dollars up front. Paradoxically, there are times when work on spec is advantageous. For example, ghostwriting for large companies or state and federal governments may be a fabulous stepping stone to regular writing contracts. Still, even when future prospects look promising, be safe rather than sorry. Always ask for *something in advance*. Notice, for example, that clause 1.1.1. (Figure 3.2) asks for a downpayment of $2,000 before your pen actually gets started. Would I accept lower? Sure, but the truth of the matter is this: paid dollars rapidly build motivation and keep your client an active part of the process.

"Can You Travel Here to Get Materials or Talk with Me?"

Frequently, over-the-telephone communication is not enough. Documents, interviews with neighbors, and just observing the client in his or her natural habitat captures critical data otherwise left to your imagination. You may be advised to personally meet the author. Travel expenses, whether you fly to the client, or the client flies to you, are entirely the client's financial responsibility. Costs incurred in any visit, from travel, lodging, meal expenses, and miscellaneous costs, are negotiated in advance before signing the contract. Even promises to repay you for your expenditures are unacceptable. For example, suppose your client asks that you make flight reservations and to be reimbursed upon your arrival. You do, figuring he or she is a trusting client.

Yes, the person may be a trusted client. But trust is only as far as you can throw a stone when it comes to new people. And this person lives, say, 1,500 miles away. Short of giving away your money for free, be stubborn. Ask that the client contact his or her own or your own travel agent, make arrangements, and then send you tickets and itinerary. Assertively protect your rights as consultant by being up front with standard travel policies. In clause 1.1.6. (Figure 4.2), note where it explicitly states that all costs are paid in advance by author by credit card or cashier's check.

"Will You Be the Spokesperson for This Book?"

Publicity scares some people. They're shy in front of cameras, hate crowds, or think they'll faint at a book signing. So, guess who they look to as an understudy? Good guess. Clients already see you as heaven sent and may beg you to represent their work beyond writing stages. Co-authorship is usually required. Ghostwriting contracts naming you as co-author naturally intensify your vested interest in the book's publishing welfare. Choice of publisher is more selective, and advances or royalty deals sweeten, knowing that a direct portion, besides agency commissions, are yours to keep. This also includes your active role in promotion after the book's release.

As promoter, trips you take outside a 100-mile radius of your locality and involving expenses for travel, lodging, and meals once again are the client's financial obligation. Determine in advance, if possible, your authorship role. If co-author, automatically assume media tours will include you. A clause such as 1.1.6.1. (see Figure 4.2) identifies the reimbursement schedule at the outset between client and independent contractor. Clarity about your public relations role and compensation schedule erases ambiguity and keeps lines of communication flowing evenly between you and client.

AUTHOR'S CORNER

"Sure," you might think, "I've recognized popular authors' names on bestseller lists, in magazine advertisements, and from small segments of radio shows during morning rush-hour driving. But, c'mon, do these people really put up with all these publishing obstacles?" Good question.

I decided to find out. Beginning in this chapter and subsequently in Chapters 5, 6, 7, and 8, results of a survey sample distributed across snail mail and e-mail are reported. Published authors (of books, software, magazines, videos, etc.) across the continental United States, whose home address, e-mail, or phone fax numbers were accessible through directories, received two correspondences. First they received a brief, friendly introduction explaining what this book was and why they were chosen as survey responders. As proof of their interest, I built in a response form that they could send back by fax, e-mail, or snail-mail affirming their willingness to participate in the survey. Responders then received a polite thank you attached to a two-page questionnaire. When I received completed questionnaires, I followed up a third and final time with a note of gratitude.

Below is a summary of questionnaire replies from book authors who kindly shared their insights, frustrations, technical information, and tips for beginning authors.

Summary of Replies from Sample Trade Book Authors in Mental Health Fields

1. **Background and degrees:** BAs in creative writing, psychology, philosophy, human services; MAs in clinical psychology, social work, nursing, journalism; PhDs in clinical psychology, organizational psychology, education.
2. **Number of books published by standard royalty publishers:** 2 to 40.
3. **Number of books published by coventure, subsidy, or other types of (self-) publishing:** 1 to 10.
4. **Average number of pages in manuscript submitted:** 360 to 500 pages.

5. **Lag time between submission and acceptance:** Some sold from proposal, some through agent, less than three months.
6. **Lag time between acceptance and publication:** 9 to 12 months.
7. **Range of advance received for acceptance:** $500 to $20,000.
8. **Range of royalty percentage received on retail or whole-sale:** 6 to 8% retail on trade paperback.
9. **Tips you offer to new writers:**

    a. Write your ideas down on paper instead of carrying them around in your head.

    b. Set regular times when you will write, getting up earlier in the day when you are fresh.

    c. Be meticulous about copyediting and proofreading. Send out clean, good-looking proposals and manuscripts.

    d. Get used to rejections.

    e. Expect revisions of your proposal and your manuscript. Nobody accepts a first draft.

RESOURCES

Publishing companies are in a constant state of flux. The first six months operating on loans are exhilarating and filled with dreams of producing the next bestseller. During this honeymoon, neophyte publishers eagerly line up printers, wholesalers, and of course their meat and potatoes—their author list. By four months into the game, still riding on the Small Business Administration (SBA) loan, the first batch of finished books is ready for the marketplace.

That's when panic strikes. One stroll through the *Publisher's Weekly* or tour through exhibits at national conferences, and reality sets in. It's a tough, competitive book-biting sales world out there. No bookseller from the megachains of Barnes & Noble to the locally owned newspaper outlets, such as Gerard News Center in Ohio, do business for nothing. They take your books if you make them money. They accept on consignment or bargain for a percentage only those books with impulse-purchase potential. Books must appear on shelves today and disappear from shelves tomorrow. If publisher X has hot books filling this need and a strong promoter to reach these outlets, they're one step higher on the survival food chain. But artsy publishers who are into esoteric, poetic works with limited market outlets may starve a while.

So, how do small "ma and pa" publishers survive the squeeze? Well, it's simple. They don't. Six months after the last bottle of champagne celebrating a new business has been poured, the publisher is filing for bankruptcy. They couldn't stay in the black. Presses with a short life span are more the rule than the exception. What keeps their finances afloat past six months is multimedia diversity and tapping into an insatiably hungry demand for books. This demand, more times than not, is for self-help, nonfiction books.

Chapter 9 contains a list of larger and smaller presses largely devoted to self-help lines of books and multimedia (CDs, audiotapes, videotapes). The list covers all areas of human services, from business to parenting to teaching behavioral tricks to pets. The publishers have been culled from several different sources or contacted directly in hopes of listing their latest accurate information and needs. As of this writing, these companies are solid revenue-producing contenders in the gallery of successful publishers. Even after this book is published, plan on 80 to 90 percent of the entries remaining in business. But, for those companies who drop out of the rat race, plan on something else–plan on their phones to be disconnected.

REFERENCES

Bintliff, R.L. (1993). *Complete manual of white-collar crime: Detection and prevention.* Englewood Cliffs, NJ: Prentice-Hall.

Corvasce, M.V. and Paglino, J.R. (1995). *Modus operandi: A writer's guide to how criminals work.* Cincinnati, OH: Writer's Digest Books.

Fowler, R.E. (1994). *The Andreasson affair.* Newberg, OR: Wildflower Press.

Keesling, B. (1996). *Sexual healing: How touch, intimacy and sexuality can heal your relationship.* Alameda, CA: Hunter House Publishers.

Keesling, B. (1996). *Sexual pleasure: Reaching new heights of sexual arousal and intimacy.* Alameda, CA: Hunter House Publishers.

McCollister, J. (1995). *Writing for dollars.* New York: Jonathan David Publishers.

Paymar, M. (1996). *Violent no more: Helping men end domestic abuse.* Alameda, CA: Hunter House Publishers.

Santrock, J., Minnett, A., and Campbell, B.D. (1994). *The authoritative guide to self-help books.* New York: Guilford Press.

Thompson, R.L. (1994). *Alien identities.* Alachua, FL: Govardhan Hill Publishing.

Tobias, M.L. and Lalich, J. (1996). *Captive hearts, captive minds: Freedom and recovery from cults and abusive relationships.* Alameda, CA: Hunter House Publishers.

Walters, E. and Walters, F. (1994). *UFO abductions in Gulf Breeze.* New York: Avon.

White-Stevens, L. (Ed.). (1996). *Hunger: The paradox of plenty.* Salt Lake City, UT: Northwest Publishing Inc.

Wilson, K.D. (1992). *Cause of death: A writer's guide to death, murder and forensic medicine.* Cincinnati, OH: Writer's Digest Books.

Wingate, A. (1992). *Scene of the crime.* Cincinnati, OH: Writer's Digest Books.

Chapter 5

Popular Magazines

Two years ago, paper prices soared to staggering record highs, draining profits from many consumer magazine publishers. Magazine industrialists got meaner, leaner, and shifted horses in midstream. Freelancer-friendly magazines, for example, turned away unsolicited articles. Publishers blamed it on a bad economy and thrifty use of in-house staff writers. As doors shut in freelancer's faces, writers either abruptly started new careers or creatively invented new opportunities for survival. They found new outlets for writing. Good writing plus perseverance and insight amazingly opened new doors, and many writers fared better than during freelancer-friendly days (Lovell, 1994; Harrop, 1995).

Now paper costs have leveled somewhat and moratoriums on hiring freelancers are removed. Still, skepticism prevails among veteran writers. They cautiously realize mainstream magazine editors are not as generous as they used to be. Stiff competition is one reason for it. More writers, sending in more proposals, forces more clever topics to be found. Bylines are harder to get. Fewer pages per magazine are available. Leftover space for freelancers is limited after advertisements and holiday promos. And why? Because of cost-cutting policies; it's reduced the number of manuscripts bought, pay rates, rights purchased, and kill fees. All of these changes figure into the diminished-space equation.

So, with editors cleaning house, is there still a viable market for mental health writers? You betcha! Nonfiction trade magazines such as *Woman's Day, Vogue, Boy's Life, Family Circle,* and *Ms.,* among others, may be budget crunchers but they have kicked up their recruitment campaigns for original contributions. The trouble is that not just any writing will do (Fredette, 1988; Friedlander and

Lee, 1995). Carefully reading *Kiwanis* magazine, for example, gives a feel for writing style, contents, and perspective. Your goal is this: find a niche within their perspective, and your rate of acceptance will be higher.

Another safe bet for niche-writing is awareness of new magazines that are directly plugged into technical and social progress. Computer and software magazines, for example, fit this description. Home-office magazines for single parents also are candy for impulse buyers.

Consumer buying trends are important to know and so we review them below. From there, feast yourself on over 200 magazines welcoming freelancer inquiries and still paying respectable compensation.

WHAT'S HOT, WHAT'S NOT

Check the temperature reading on your local newsstand. It's sizzling. Colorfully printed headlines race across the page arousing your curiosity. *Aliens attack at night!* Now that sounds intriguing, eh? When nobody is looking, you nonchalantly pick up the magazine and flip through it. You're dying to find out when the aliens attacked and where they did it. Face it, you're a glutton for tabloid smut. You turn right to the feature story and snort in all of the sensationalistic details you can

Consumer magazines flirt with everybody's inner lust for public obscenity. Even conservative rags such as *Redbook* stir potent fantasies in true-confession stories on intimacy, infidelity, and secret lovemaking. All topics, all stories, and every cover smacks a bit of perversion. Mastheads artistically can dazzle your eyes, and emotionally seductive titles such as "I Trusted Him and He Raped Me" (Dolgoff, 1996) electrically charge an irresistible visual magnet. You can't pull yourself away from it.

Today's magazine covers, like their contents, heavily focus on instant gratification. Editors know that the average buyer peruses several magazines within minutes. Seconds later, the competition is over, and frequently there's only one winner. Winners have headlines and articles aggressively shouting out morally reprehensible ideas surrounded by sordid or overly explicit pictures, and graphics, all calibrated to grab your attention. And, it works. Perhaps readers are gullible or simply want escape from their mundane lives. For whatever reason, effective magazine advertising begins and ends with covers and articles depicting the cesspool of human morbidity.

That is why writing for magazines is not a scholarly task. It's an exercise in pure people-watching. Know the people, culture, and their taste in mental stimulation, and the rest is easy. Selecting a topic is facile after sizing up your audience. Think in terms of "grocery-shop mentality" for a frame of reference. Saturday and Sunday morning shoppers are predominantly your first line of readers. Now, choose from the list below for subjects. These topics represent 90 percent of readers' choices from a cross-section of consumer magazines.

Self-Help

General how-to articles provide needed relief from painfully boring work schedules and single lifestyles. Singles are a statistically growing majority. Young people enter the workforce earlier and stay single longer. Single parents frequently struggle to raise children without child support dollars and endlessly juggle between nurturing others and themselves. Without partners, personal problems rest entirely on their own shoulders. Household chores, financial decisions, vacation and recreational choices, even cooking hints for three-minute meals are everyday obstacles. Articles addressing these problems in simple-to-use solutions are long-awaited answers to a prayer.

Take, for instance, "Please Don't Hit Your Kids" (LeShan, 1996). Author of 27 books, Eda LeShan has reassuring advice for spiteful parents intolerant of their "brats." Anita Cheng's "Why Do I Hate My Job?" (1996) also offers a calming panacea for work hostility. And time-management expert Franny Van Nevel unravels the self-destructive pace of busy women in her "One-Hour Organizers" (1996). Each of these articles affectionately treats a defeating habit and inspires a quick rebound for healthier growth. Readers thrive on self-help advice since it replaces costly therapy and unwanted criticism from friends or parents.

Vanity

Indulge your voyeuristic fantasies for a moment. Imagine getting an authorized glimpse of the beauty world's hired guns. Exclusive access to supermodels: Chanel's Kirsty Hume, Clairol's Linda Evangelista, Revlon's Cindy Crawford, Cover Girl's Niki Taylor, and Estee Lauder's Elizabeth Hurley. Alone at last in a private boutique, you get their full and undivided attention as each reveals intimate secrets. Sound enticing?

For some, maybe. Some men and women are so vain, that they simply gush for details on supermodels' lifestyles. Articles on vanity focus on self-beautification ranging from diets to aerobics to cosmetics to fashion. Self-perfection is a recurrent underlying theme. Dress smart, plaster on an award-winning smile, routinely eat Slim Fast bars for lunch, and you've just about reached Nirvana. Ultimate self-actualization, readers believe, comes from polishing their outward persona. Too much polishing, says Laurie Tarkan in "The Dangers of Dieting" (1996) is poisoning your emotional wellness. So, too, does overdoing apparel. It bleaches out the honesty and emotional self-love you deserve—just ask Rebecca Ascher-Walsh in "Dress Down, Stand Tall" (1996).

Obsession with purifying oneself is both fortified and defused in vanity articles. Choose the perspective you feel a calling for. Sad to say, choosing the ethically healthy standpoint—defusing bad habits—doesn't sell well. Cash registers ring frequently when advice motivates high energy self-indulgence.

Love and Sex

Did you know pumpkin pie and lavender cause penile engorgement? That chocolate is forbidden some in convents? These chemical aphrodisiacs, among other discoveries tying biology to sexuality, sprung forth with Dr. Crenshaw's book *The Alchemy of Love and Lust* (1996). Body-sending messages of love and romance are only one example of the prolific books and magazine articles exploiting love and sex for mass consumption. Themes revolve largely around (a) dating couples, (b) marriage and romance, (c) sexual enhancers, (d) gender role dominance, and (e) testimonials revealing unrelented secrets of infidelity.

Consider, for example, Joy Davidson's "When He Wants Her to Play Eliza to His Professor Higgins" (1996). Here she pokes fun at monopolizing males suffering superiority complexes. Dating Mr. or Mrs. Right, says author Rebecca Cutter (1996a; 1996b) is a matter of "opposites attracting." Even when face-to-face matchmaking is impractical, take Linda Gross' advice on joining the video revolution in "Video Dating: What to Expect" (1996). Or, take a familiar road to heightened sexuality. Begin at home with your spouse. Eileen Livers reminds you to "Seduce Your Husband: What Works and What Backfires" (1996).

Of course, oversolicitous seductions may not just backfire, but can build up his expectations of your sexual assertiveness while he remains cold, insensitive, and demanding. That's what Michael Segell's "The Unfeeling Brute" (1996) warns women. Still, heterosexual love and heartbreak only represents half the literature. Extensive readership looks for articles on gay and lesbian romance, such as James Hardy's "When Love Hurts: Male on Male Abuse in the Gay Culture" (1996a) and *B-Boy Blues* (1996b).

In all, articles read best when they integrate contemporary themes such as AIDS, rape, dating, and divorce with innovative new angles showing villain, victim, and of course, ultimate victory.

Money and Power

Success sagas are the main course for working singles aspiring for career advancement and self-discipline. Insightful tips on overcoming workplace traps, on budgeting for rainy days, layoffs, and downsizing, and for building a nest egg while young, all comprise the practical how-to articles on what money and power can do for you. Articles take two perspectives. The first are litmus tests of consumer growth indexes. Articles address rising debts, interests rates, mortgages, stock options, borrowing binges, and resisting credit card companies who offer enticements. Money management using prudent thinking dominates this discussion.

A second genre of articles profiles enterprising shakers and movers and celebrity heroes of success. Articles stress upwardly mobile lifestyles and how to perfect job interviews. Nancy Austin's "The New Job Interview: Beyond the Trick Question" (1996) is a good example. Rising to success also entails making prudent financial decisions and learning to live within moderate means. Still, not all articles are heavy downers on being conservative accountants. Celebrity interviews in, for example, *Style* magazine, give readers a privileged peak behind closed doors of rich and famous people from Steven Spielberg to Microsoft mogul Bill Gates, now rated the richest man in the world.

Well-known stars such as Tom Cruise and Brad Pitt always make wonderful profiles. Or, be courageous. Try interviewing movie and TV's high-salary newcomers who combine acting and good looks: seek interviews with Kyra Sedgwick (*Phenomenon*), Matthew McConaughey (*A Time to Kill*), Billy Crudup (*Everyone Says I Love You*), Skeet Ulrich (*Albino Alligator*), and Edward Norton (*The People vs. Larry Flynt*).

Cyberspace and Computer Gizmos

Blasting into today's world of cyberpunks and adult computer junkies are hundreds of how-to, practical articles on effectively browsing the internet. Readers have unquenchable thirsts for updated World Wide Web sights, latest hardware, software, and accessory gadgets, and tipsters' do's and don'ts on breaking into protected files. Adored shopping sites and trusted web resources, for example, are a regular department for *The Net: The Ultimate Internet Guide*, an avant-garde magazine, only in its second year, which has already quadrupled its subscription, number of pages, and high-paying advertising space. And why? Because it completely delivers what readers want: the hottest technology for a surfing edge over other net users.

Even company magazines such as *Adobe Magazine* have gotten into the act. Adobe's monthly magazine originally was a showcase for purely Adobe products. But times have changed. Now it is a marketplace for other internet toys. Not just current toys, but toys in the future. *Make your own CD* is ahead for future cybersleuths and can be followed in article after article, describing this technology's rise to commercial availability.

What makes computer articles so voluptuous are two factors: supply and demand. Here's the demand: Computers are not what they used to be. Rapidly increasing techno operations from higher-speed modems to interactive devices and simplified installation and repairs, such as do-it-yourself insertable gigabyte drives and troubleshooting communication errors, all have put consumers in the driver's seat. No longer the passive bystander, today's highly sophisticated user knows what he or she wants, and wants it now. Demand is for immediate supplies.

The MacDonalds' "fast-food" mentality has adults wanting childish instant gratification. And most computer vendors fully intend to meet this demand. But software solutions cannot stand alone. They require accompanying articles and books sorting through the morass of information overload. That way, "make-me-feel-good" users are happy with their purchases and in time will be addictively hooked into buying more products.

Weird, X-Files, and Alien Abductions

Ufologists and lay skywatchers alike not only contribute mega-bucks to trade book sales but are consummate magazine subscribers. They line up in droves for the monthly editions of *UFO Sightings*. Bolstering this E.T. epidemic are widely circulating news stories on the paranormal, alien abductions, crop circles, telekinesis, and radio transmitter implantations. TV docudramas such as *Sightings, Encounters,* and *Unsolved Mysteries* project realism in reportings of firsthand accounts, while personifying life beyond the stars as explorable and attainable.

Unlike "Trekkies," cult followers are not necessarily science-fiction buffs. Professionals such as psychologists, laboratory microbiologists, chemists, even eminent scholars in astronomy have secret passions for space travel, alien contact, and discovery of governmentally suppressed information. Nobody is spared the driving impetus for coveted knowledge.

Authors seriously addressing this phenomenon should first read a few articles. Note that discussions distinctly contain empirical documentation along with testimonials. Retrospective interviews of abductees and spaceship photographers accompany proof of their claims either in figures (e.g., photographs, drawings) or in tables (tabulated data from interview studies). Clinical reports of abductees under hypnosis may include session transcripts with analytical commentary. Rarely are there purely hypothetical pontifications in print. Everything has some factual support. Speculation is one thing;

but most guesswork is derivative of whatever "scientific data" has been collected, described, and offered as legitimate evidence.

Wholesome Family

With a reading culture inundated by space aliens, explosive computer technology, and sexual obsessions, is there any room left for "I love my family" literature? Sure, why not? Mama Bear and Papa Bear stories capture Americana in magazines on genealogy, reunions, camping, and apple-pie baking traditions. Still popular, editor-friendly trades gaining subscription speed are *Family Motor Coaching, Country Woman, Better Homes and Gardens*, and *Camping Today*. These magazines present sentimental reminders of family picnics, wholesome fun, and uncomplicated lifestyles. In a Norman Rockwell picturesque way, articles stress parental love, renewal of forgotten crafts (weaving, crocheting), mealtime preparations (back to meat and potatoe), and ways to preserve treasures of family legacies.

JOURNALISM 101

How many written words does it take to say "love?" Compassion, romance, friendship, trust, sex, intimacy–each a slight variation of the other but conveying a uniform meaning: feelings. Feeling words are holograms of inner human expression. They symbolically transcend inner emotions into written words that are read and understood, we hope, by readers who can translate the message. Accurately encoded messages get our ideas across. Inaccurate translations do the opposite; readers think they know but really have no idea what we said.

And so the real art of magazine writing lies in Journalism 101. That is, in expressing your thoughts rapidly and easily. No jargon. No legal, bureaucratic, or technical terminology. Nothing ornate. This will only confuse readers and obscure meanings (Cook, 1996; Mears, 1995). Write just the facts and just the feelings. Include informal chit-chat style, using short sentences, few dangling modifiers, and short, easy-to-read words. While sounding simple enough, journalistic writing is a tough change for academic pros.

In scholarly writing, conventions dictate using technical terms, colloquial phrases, and smartly talking in third-person voice (e.g., "a group of rats was examined that . . . "). Personalizing discussion of things you actually did is taboo. Sure, take credit, but do so in a pluralistic way (e.g., "our results showed that . . . "). Academic styles also require support for your beliefs. "UFOs are invading the planet," just doesn't cut it. Whereas, based on your research you might say, "evidence of extraplanetary visits was shown by collecting such and such data." Validity and reliability of your claims is a must. You *must* properly follow the canons of good scientific and scholarly writing by documenting creative ideas.

But not in magazine writing. Documentation is important but not essential. Opinions must be credible, referring to some study or evidence. But spare the reader gross details of whether data were quantitative or qualitative. Write just the facts and keep it organized in a fashion understood by a reader with an eighth-grade reading level (Wilson, 1993; Yudkins, 1993). Here are some other hints for preparing your first draft:

1. Use metaphors.
2. Write short sentences.
3. Use short, punchy words.
4. Feature one idea per paragraph.
5. Use real examples.

Use Metaphors

Metaphors, sure, are colorful words–words typically used in another context taking on new meaning for a stronger mental picture in the reader's mind. For example, you start with "His anger was violently aggressive and powerfully intimidating." Now, let's revise this phrase and add an animal metaphor to it: "His anger was lionlike in its ferocity." Lions, we know, have a ferocious growl. Fierce kings of the jungle are predatory and act superior over smaller animals. Even in animated Disney movies, lions command an unchallenged throne over other beasts. So, in one word, you instantly picture a source of powerful aggression without ever using the words "power" and "aggression."

Metaphors also are valuable in titles. Take, for instance, *The soul of a new machine*. Notice "soul" doubles in meaning. It means the inner wiring of computers and heartbeat of today's modern computer compared to future models. News writing frequently does this, for example, *Broadway wraps on high note*. Here reports of theatrical box office receipts for fiscal 1995 are impressive, especially the increased ticket sales for musicals. "High notes" plays on the theme of musicals.

Write Short Sentences

Divide sentences as you've never done before. Feature one simple idea for each sentence. Keep dangling modifiers to a minimum. Instead of saying, *They arrived under the auspices of the companies they represent, many of whom were Fortune 500, all struggling with downsizing*, chop it in half and leave out additive phrases. Smooth it over to read as, *They arrived under the auspices of the companies they represent. These Fortune 500 companies all struggled with downsizing.*

That doesn't mean make sentences boring. Creatively flavor your sentences with colons, semicolons, hyphens, and quoted material. That way, ancillary thoughts are inserted without distracting the readers. For example, notice a variety of grammatical shifts while creating a sensual mood: *Her beauty radiated luminously—but beauty was also skin deep. Her personal and business side was ravishing; every inch of her career ambition drew envy from my lips.*

Use Short, Punchy Words

Punchy words are not a hard and fast rule. In fact, few rigid rules apply to magazine composition. But one unwritten rule frequently followed is what advertisers have known for years: catapult your ideas with jack-in-the-box words and phrases. In *Daily Variety*, for example—probably the best punchy writing around—feel the electrical voltage rushing through this movie reviewer's opening lines:

Sports comedies are inherently predictable, but this fantasy, about a fan who winds up head coach of an NBA team, seems especially uninspired. Whoopi Goldberg's wholehearted and likable performance, while occasionally funny, is simply not enough to lead this standard-issue programmer to victory. The third basketball film to be released in five weeks—after box office airballs *Celtic Pride* and *Sunset Park*—*Eddie* will likely be sent to the showers early in its theatrical run. (Hindes, 1996, p. 4)

One Idea Per Paragraph

Pace your material so that only one idea occurs in a paragraph. Paragraphs can be short, from one to three sentences, rather than drag on for pages. Orations, in other words, are out of the question. Even a one-word sentence linked together by chains of semicolons and hyphens is catchy. *The rank odor of dog litter permeated the room—but nobody claimed responsibility for the filthy mess; that meant Harold was in trouble.*

Use Real Examples

Writing for consumers is a personal invitation into their world. Your writing periscope gets a peek at lifestyles of Mr. and Mrs. Average. That's where your examples come from. Think of how comedians do it: you think up stupid, ridiculous, and humiliating experiences everybody experiences on a daily or weekly basis. Choose from this array of fruitful samples, cleverly illustrating your ideas.

Take, for example, parenting. See if you can vicariously relate to this story. *My two-year old dragged a dusty stuffed animal out of the attic and into his fresh, clean sheets. That annoyed me. I just changed his sheets not an hour ago. But I kept my cool. With a slight diversion, and no yelling and screaming, I pulled it off. Mr. Teddy Bear's outing was cut short. I got rid of it. And Junior didn't even know the difference.*

AUTHOR'S CORNER

Below is a summary of questionnaire replies from magazine authors who kindly shared their insights, frustrations, technical information, and tips for beginning authors.

Summary of Replies from Sample Consumer Magazine Writers in Mental Health and Allied Fields

1. **Background and degrees:** BAs in sociology, psychology, business, education, English, journalism, broadcasting, editing; MAs in clinical psychology, social work, journalism, history; PhDs in clinical psychology (few PhDs)
2. **Number of articles published in magazines:** 5 to 100
3. **Number of articles dealing with mental health:** 1 to 25; areas of lifestyle, personal need, profiles, self-improvement, culture, dance, vehicular safety, fitness, self-realization, dating
4. **Average number of words per manuscript:** 1,000 to 5,000 words
5. **Lag time between submission and acceptance:** 3 to 4 weeks to 3.5 years
6. **Names of magazines you've published in recently:** *Heartland USA, Working Woman, Executive Female, Country America, Equus, Florida Living, Accent, Better Homes & Gardens, USA Weekend, Chicago Sun Times, Hollywood Reporter, Golden Years, Family Circle, Cigar Afficionado, The Economist, Car & Driver, Newsweek, Time, Off Duty, Today's Black Woman, Woman's World, Sassy, Mademoiselle, Woman's Day, McCall's, Self, Just Seventeen, Your Health, Cosmopolitan, Parenting, Working Mother*
7. **Range of pay for manuscripts:** $0.50 to $0.90/per word; $100 to $2,000 outright purchase
8. **Do you do more writing by assignment?** Sixty percent indicated getting editor's approval first; 20 percent said they prepare and submit articles on spec or without prior editorial approval; 20 percent said they do both
9. **Tips offered to new writers:**

   a. Never, ever give up.
   b. Write concisely.
   c. Know the magazine and its audience.
   d. Humor sells.
   e. Don't be afraid to overedit.
   f. Emphasize the business end of writing.
   g. Sharpen your writing craft.

h. Figure out the editorial slant either by reading the magazine or asking for editorial guidelines.
i. Be specific in a pitch; explain how you would make it interesting and timely.
j. Use colorful examples to avoid dreary dullness.
k. Never be deflated by personalized rejections. Regard it as a compliment that somebody actually looked at your manuscript.
l. Seek the scores of outlets for publishing instead of putting your eggs in one basket.
m. Don't undersell yourself. Ask for reasonable dollars for hard labor.
n. Try to recycle the same story with different angles for multiple sales.
o. Remember that editors are busy and they receive many calls. Make your pitch a memorable one.
p. Always do your homework by first understanding a magazine's needs. Never call up an editor cold asking what they need. It really annoys him or her.
q. Agent or no agent, the person who can really make things happen is yourself.

RESOURCES

Sure, magazine freelancing seems outlandish. Think about it. Can you believe you're being paid to write an article? Probably the last time you wrote articles and got them published was for academic journals. Remember how great you felt once you received your acceptance letter. "I did it! I passed the grueling peer-referred process!" Kudos for your efforts. But no matter how high you felt seeing your paper months later in print, it didn't pay the rent. Payment for writing academic articles? I don't think so.

Well, at least that used to be true. The practice of noncompensation for academic writing is itself in transition, with many esteemed journals (e.g., APA periodicals) following fast the leads of their paying, commercial counterparts. Now scholarly authors can get a dime or two for publishing some research articles. So, who knows, by 2001, perhaps published advice will have a price tag well worth the time and energy to write the article.

Until then, academic-turned-popular writers are in competition with nonhuman-service writers who have mastered the art of fact-finding and speed writing for big bucks. They already have the process of pitching, writing on assignment, and knowing what the magazine wants down to a pure science. They've almost cornered the market entirely. So, with this bottleneck in freelancing, why enter the crowded traffic?

I'll tell you why. Credentials. It's always credentials. Your degree, training, and expertise is a commodity more precious than diamonds. On the stockmarket of author trading, that MA or PhD after your name pays a high dividend for editors who know their readers want facts from authorities. And that's where you come in.

Author credentials carry a distinction, drawing immediate attention if the topic you propose is relevant and fits the magazine's focus. Well-written articles fitting a niche always will clobber a wannabe mental health expert who is really a journalist in disguise. And, of course, given a couple of years' worth of writing for magazines under your belt, you'll have the best of both worlds. You'll be a freelancer whiz at composing timely pieces, who has the encyclopedic knowledge of human behavior.

That leads us to magazine resources. The resources listed in Chapter 9 are only paying magazines. They run the gamut from sports to animal training.

REFERENCES

Ascher-Walsh, R. (1996). Dress Down, Stand Tall. *McCalls*, April, pp. 50-53.

Austin, N. (1996). The New Job Interview: Beyond the Trick Question. *Working Woman*, March, pp. 23-24.

Cheng, A. (1996). Why Do I Hate My Job? *Mademoiselle*, April, p. 34.

Cook, M.J. (1996). *Leads and conclusions*. Cincinnati, OH: Writer's Digest Books.

Crenshaw, T. (1996). *The alchemy of love and lust*. New York: Putnam Books.

Cutter, R. (1996a). Opposites Attract. *Woman's Own*, April, pp. 34-35.

Cutter, R. (1996b). *When opposites attract: Right brain/left brain relationships and how to make them work*. New York: Dutton.

Davidson, J. (1996). When He Wants Her to Play Eliza to His Professor Higgins, *Cosmopolitan*, March, pp. 106-109.

Dolgoff, S. (1996). I Trusted Him and He Raped Me. *Young and Modern,* March, pp. 75-77

Fredette, J.M. (Ed.). (1988). *Handbook of magazine article writing.* Cincinnati, OH: Writer's Digest Books.

Friedlander, E.J. and Lee, J. (1995). *Feature writing for newspapers and magazines: The pursuit of excellence.* New York: HarperCollins College.

Gross, L. (1996). Videodating: What to Expect. *Woman's Own,* April, pp. 95-97.

Hardy, J.E. (1996a). When Love Hurts: Male on Male Abuse in the Gay Culture. *Men's Style,* March, pp. 35, 38.

Hardy, J.E. (1996b). *B-boy blues.* New York: Alyson Publications.

Harrop, T. (1995). *Getting published: An insider's guide to creating you first break in magazine writing.* New York: Whitefish Editions.

Hindes, A. (1996). *Eddie:* Film review. *Daily Variety,* May 31, (4), 31.

LeShan, E. (1996). Please Don't Hit Your Kids. *Mademoiselle,* April, pp. 40-43.

Livers, E. (1996). Seduce your Husband: What Works and What Backfires. *McCall's,* April, pp. 114, 116.

Lovell, R. (1994). *Freelancing: A guide to writing for magazines and other markets.* New York: Waveland Press.

Mears, W.R. (1995). *The new news business.* New York: HarperPerennial.

Segell, M. (1996). The Unfeeling Brute. *Esquire,* March, pp. 65-67.

Tarkan, L. (1996). The Dangers of Dieting. *McCall's,* April, pp. 110-112.

VanNevel, F. (1996). One Hour Organizers. *Woman's Day,* April, pp. 30, 34.

Wilson, J. (1993). *The complete guide to magazine article writing.* Cincinnati, OH: Writer's Digest Books.

Yudkins, M. (1993). *Freelance writing for magazines and newspapers.* New York: HarperCollins.

Chapter 6

Software Companies

Designing your own software is an intriguing endeavor usually dominated by computer technicians. Ten years ago, when industry watchers predicted programmers would be the next superior race, software developers belonged to an exclusive group. They were the only ones who knew "technical hieroglyphics." They would hide early in the morning and late at night in computer labs, rarely showing their faces. Nobody knew them, but they existed. Likened to experimental psychologists, innately talented computer engineers lead a discrete life romantically bonded to their digital machines.

Using complex binary codes, software developers designed programs that opened up, ran smoothly, and politely closed. Rarely, if ever, did users really know how this occurred. It didn't matter. All that mattered is that the program worked. Little did we users know what lay underneath the surface of PC magic. Running a word processor, spread sheet, or any other program was a circuitry of calculated information linking segments of operation together. Original computer languages such as Basic, FORTRAN, and Cobalt, and new generations of systems called C++, Visual Basic, Visual Foxpro, Object-Vision, and Java made our life easier. Each had its own toolchest of configurations uniquely tuned for faster, more comprehensive performance. So, for years, we never questioned what computer doctors were doing in surgery. Conceptually or practically, understanding computer anatomy was over our heads. That was then.

Today, computer surgery is open to all of us. Even the term programming is archaic. Now it's called "software authoring." Products enabling noncomputer analysts to write fairly intelligible programs for daily application are available and widely popular.

With simple instructions, any user can assemble an elementary string of commands and see the results in seconds. And that's only the beginning. How about programming ideas? Hundreds of software games, graphics, office accessories, and writing tools started as a concept. Somewhere, a dream team brainstorms software ideas from germinal stages until the program reaches market maturity.

Who does this? Well, you can. National software giants such as Adobe and Microsoft may have their own creative departments, but your input is precisely what their creative departments seek in consumer product viability. Smaller software producers rely more heavily on consumer suggestions since they target specific market groups and want to sell products that buyers prefer.

You're not only a buyer, you're also an insightful observer of human systems and can size up potential software directions of great interest to companies. In this chapter, you'll see just exactly how a brilliant idea for software can proceed from a mental picture to manufacturing (Dewitt, 1989). Either you can spearhead the entire process, marketing and selling your products, or you can find a software publisher who will do it for you. In either case, earning dollars from software creation opens new doors of opportunity.

WHAT'S HOT, WHAT'S NOT

Just as books and magazines have lucrative themes, so the software industry hustles their best-selling products for megadollars. Let's explore a sampling of these prize winners for a course on how to begin.

Games

Let me tell you about games. There was a time when Sega and Atari were kingpins of interactive electrical toys. They usurped the reigning powers of pinball machines and video arcades. Children ages 6 to 16 stayed home hypnotically entranced in Mario Brothers and Ninja Turtle adventures, outsmarting video opponents by how cleverly they manipulated buttons, switches, and levers. Then, five years later, a more advanced intellectual challenge arrived on the scene, teasing both memory and visual motor coordination. That challenge was complex graphic software games featuring semireal-istic voices, animations, and gorgeous 3-D graphics. Games were faster, action was more exciting, and enemy forces were meaner, more diabolical, and compelling to destroy. The games featured planet empires battling it out, warlords demolishing civilization, and flight and military simulations overriding your reality.

High-tech software games are engrossing. You clearly must be a seasoned programmer to write one, but not to create one. Powerful games never truly saturate the market. They remain in constant demand. Your creative mind may latch onto an idea based on some observant trends in child and teen cultures, such as games involving rollerblades or internet mysteries. Invent the concept first and worry less about how this invention can materialize.

Virtual Reality

What do *Lawnmower Man* and *Virtuosity* have in common? Transformation in space and time. That's the ultimate simulation artificially created using virtual reality (VR). Commercial VR prod-ucts are still a high-price item but slowly are becoming affordable. Within five years, a visual headset (now about $300 to $1,000) and VR software running on Windows 95 or Macintosh will entice a fantasy-seeking public beyond imagination. As developers hurry toward the madness of the Christmas buying season, VR ideas pay a premium. VR products typically focus on sensory stimulation. Walking, flying, driving, fighting, or moving rapidly through space guarantees an adrenaline rush entirely driven by computer imagery. Can you come up with an idea using sensory input? I believe you can.

Sex

Sex is hot, but it always has been. Produce a series of games, raunchier than the rest, and you've got yourself a million-dollar, runaway hit. Why? Because sex has alluring value. Adult sex soft-ware programs are analogs of sensuous talk and risky encounters most users would be terrified of pursuing outside of their computer

world. But secretly they can have a steamy affair with the body-per-
fect gender of their choice. Then, as the game begins, they have
role-playing exchanges likened to a bar scene.

In one game called *Midnight Stranger,* for example, you choose
your hangout spot, from corner cafe to disco. Inside, you're greeted
by males or females inviting you over for a closer look. On the
screen below these people is a panel you click if you want your
reply either to sound soft and flirtatious or insulting and belligerent.
In response, the near graphically perfect man or woman is more
solicitous or tells you to go away. It's quite absorbing.

Computer-generated liaisons are purely for entertainment. While
practitioners may argue they have therapeutic value, as in teaching
social skills, therapy is quickly overshadowed by competition.
Users treat sex games equal to empire-destroyer games insofar as
rushing to score the highest points in the shortest amount of time.
Writing proposals for sex games should seriously consider another
point. Dating a computer-simulated partner is light years from realistic dating. You can calibrate, control, and predict computer
answers that rapidly build up your masculine or feminine esteem.
But apply this temple of esteem in real-world encounters, where
chance replaces control, and watch the temple pillars of esteem
crumble in seconds.

An ingenious alternative, then, may be a sex game incorporating
realistic situations and didactics for, say, high schoolers or premari-
tal adults on how to curb their own promiscuity or refuse sexual
advances. Ideas flourish when you employ clinical observations
into game-like scenarios. I know you can do that.

Edutainment

"Edutainment" is the assimilation of two themes in software
games: education and entertainment. The purpose is to make learning fun. Games of this caliber are less speedtraps and more geared
for informing users on particular topics. Multimedia CDs and software such as the Encyclopedia Britannica feature combined sound
and graphic files for a spectacular tour through knowledge. Plane-
tary and astronomy software have video files of footage taken from
the Hubbell telescope or vintage clips of Apollo and Columbia
shuttle launches. Even typing-tutor software includes video files

(AVI) and sound files (WAV) that open up as rewards for mastering new levels of difficulty.

Edutainment is clearly *the* market for young minds who represent tomorrow's digital revolution. A learning tool that combines sound and video has unlimited sales potential for teachers, parents, and kids.

The Four F's: Fast, Furious, Far-Out, Fun

In general, any software idea twirling around in your mind must meet the four "F's." It must be *fast, furious, far-out,* and *fun.* Games with speed attract players with "jet-ski" mentalities who are rush seekers and thrive on rising challenges of skill and luck. Furious games never are frustrating. They drive a dual dose of fear and intrigue into players aspiring for "rock'em, sock'em" interaction with simulated monsters, warlords, beasts, or enemy fighter ships they can laser into oblivion.

Far-out games tickle their fancy for outrageous fantasy. Space travel into distant galaxies is one way. Encounters with paranormal species or ghostly phenomena are another. But even normal or terrestrial settings with a highly ingenious twist count as far-out. Take, for example, a Nazi hunt game where you and your bayonet start off in a castle and end up high above the clouds in mid-air pursuit of the enemy.

Finally, it must be fun. Exciting software, whether for serious or recreational players, has enough multimedia effects that make it hard to log off. Hours are spent visually gorging your creative mind and skillfully testing your abilities. Meet these basic criteria, and your software developing days have begun.

Here Today and Gone Tomorrow

One other fascinating rule about software development is this: there's never enough. Computer upgrades in speed (megahertz), in memory (RAM), in storage (MB), and in operating systems (e.g., Windows 95, Power Macintosh) are so constant that software must keep up with the rat race. Ten years ago, DOS-run systems crudely limited versatility in software for IBM users.

Today, with Windows 95, processing speed is light years beyond DOS and capable of running far faster and more complex, multimedia software for IBM and IBM compatible computers. Software that lags behind this advancing progress in computers becomes obsolete. Unlike classic books, which never die, there is no classic software. Software dies and gets buried in no time.

Software with a short shelf life sells well. Reordered stock is usually never a problem within a reasonable period of months. But beyond those months, the software already is back in service being upgraded. Think about the word processing software you have. You probably purchased it years ago when it was a "1.0" version. Now, years later, assuming it functions on advanced computer models, repeated upgrades market it as "6.0." In other words, it didn't stay static. Market survival meant improving its performance.

DO YOU NEED TO BE A COMPUTER GENIUS?

Is there an art to talking in computer language? My wife does it with extraordinary eloquence. I don't. Technical jargon is impressive and instantly builds a fraternal bond with programmers who think you're one of them. But, you're not, so don't fake it. Learn, like most of us do, that effective software proposals can be in simple English. You can describe sequences of action, as presented in Chapter 3. Talking in programming lingo is less important than knowing exactly how you expect the computer to generate your ideas. Computer literacy helps you do that. Know, for instance, how to operate CDs, how wave and video files open and the mechanisms to create them. Your experience using multimedia digital programs on making movies (sound, video, pictures, morphing, etc.), scanning pictures, and even surfing on-line servers all contribute to polished proposals.

SOFTWARE AUTHORING PROGRAMS

By now, you've probably caught the message of this book: join the do-it-yourself bandwagon. Clinicians, trainers, planners, administrators are all seeking financially expedient ways of reaching learners. Traditionally, access was through books, videos, audiotapes, even direct workshops. These are still effective outlets, but not in the computer industry. Whether learners are buyers, patients, or employees, software development is rapidly shifting in one major direction: writing and programming are done in-house. That's given birth to author-software programs.

Multimedia authoring programs help you create computer-based training and presentations that harness text, audio, graphics, and even video. While not a substitute for products out of high-tech computer labs, authoring software offers a simpler tool for interactive programs using what is called "hyperlink." In a nutshell, here's the advantages of what you'll get:

1. It provides multimedia developers built-in paradigms or models for setting up learning models and entertainment.
2. Complexity is at your discretion. Some software contains complex scripting-based applications giving your creativity unlimited freedom. Or, play it easy and confine your choices to one or two methods or systems.
3. It offers an efficiently faster method of programming without hours spent on telephone conferences with "real programmers."

Selecting a Software Tool

Where do you begin? Experts say there are no simple rules for selecting author software. Authoring tools vary too much in their design and use. But, in cost-conscious times, clinical software shoppers want help narrowing down the vast array of choices faced on the shelf. Consider, as helpers, the following six guidelines to authoring software selection.

Select a Tool That Suits Your Technical Ability

Software should be easy to use and have simple directions for interface, that is, how you can integrate it with other communication devices and networks. Two interfaces to choose from are "language-based" and "menu-based." Language-based interfaces let you create exactly what you want but only if you're literate in computer programming. Oh well, forget that one.

Menu-based interfaces, for us nonprogrammers, prompt you through easy-to-follow steps to create training, educational, and treatment objectives.

Make Sure the Authoring Software Has All the Key Linking and Performance Features

Software features should allow you to at least present information, ask questions, judge answers, branch back and forth from ideas and lessons, and save data about your own or another person's behavior. Failure in these capacities means the software requires links with additional hardware or software, for a price, of course.

Understand How the Product Is Priced and Look for Hidden Costs

Notice in Table 6.1 the average authoring software price is $300 to $500, with some prices towering in the upper thousands. Fees also are paid for each person who uses the software. This is how user-licenses work. Software companies may either sell you a "site-license," covering all users at the site, or a "per-user license," where a surcharge is on each person expected to use your program.

Still a third penalty for using authoring software involves fees charged for every copy of the training program you create with their product. Called "runtime fees," connecting this software to other software packages is copying the proprietary software. You unfortunately can't give away their product or derivatives of their product for free—even if you've paid a steep purchase price.

Determine How Much Help You Will Get from the Software Itself or from the Supplier

Products vary in terms of support hotlines for help. Manuals, of course, make meager efforts at answering the most *frequently asked questions* (FAQ). But, as you have discovered, what others frequently ask never is what you ask. Check with company representa-

TABLE 6.1. Multimedia authoring software programs

Software	Requires	Price	Contact
Allegiant Supercard	Mac/Power PC	$595	Allegiant Technologies 619-587-0500
Media Wrangler	Windows	$99	AltaVista Technologies 408-364-8777
The Instructor	Windows Windows 95	$795	BCD Associates 406-843-4574
Design-a-Course	Windows Windows 95	$175-$473	Bernstein & Associates 800-511-5299
Course Builder Total Solution	Windows Windows 95 Mac/Power PC	$995	Discovery Systems International 423-690-8829
SuperLink Plus	Windows Windows 95	$400	DSP Solutions 415-919-4000
Special Delivery	Mac/Power PC	$259	Interactive Media Corp. 415-948-0745
Testmaster	Windows	$299	InterCom 800-298-7070
MediaDeveloper	Windows Windows 95	$495	Lenel Systems International 716-248-9720
Media Verse	Windows Windows 95	$749	Looking Glass Software 310-348-8240
HyperWriter 4.2 for Training	Windows	$995	Ntergaid Incorporation 203-783-1283
Expo 1.0	Windows Windows 95	$399	Paul Mace Software 503-488-2322
Act II Multimedia Authoring System	DOS	$495	Performance Software Inc 203-953-4040
Learning Processor	Windows Windows 95	$995	Pinnacle Multimedia 801-562-5900
SoftBook Maker	Windows Windows 95	$499	Softbooks Inc. 714-586-1284
Learning Master Toolkit 1.1	Mac/Power PC	$149	Systran, Inc. 713-480-8004
Tutor-Teach	Windows Mac/Power PC	$99	Techware Corporation 800-347-3224
Videodisc Authoring Toolkit	Mac/Power PC	$450	Video Image Presentation Systems 714-951-9169
Cinemation 1.1	Mac/Power PC	$295	Vividus Corporation 415-321-2221

tives before buying the product. Do they have on-line help? Is support built into the program to help you understand various confusing features? Whether by telephone, electronic bulletin board, or help menus within the program, rapid access to consulting relieves aggravation and provides needed tips for running the software.

Double Check the Technical Specifications of the Hardware and the Operating System

Strange, you may say, but frequently software is bought without first checking if it meets your computer "specs." Authoring systems you select may have fabulous crystals of magic but be inoperable on your Macintosh. Ask yourself if your own computer or computers you expect to run this software on are compatible with operating requirements of the program. If it absolutely runs on Windows 95, Macintosh (Mac) is out. Mac is in and IBMs are history if the software is only Macintosh friendly.

Try Before You Buy

Do you ever try on clothing before you say, "Okay, I'll buy it." Of course you do. Expensive computer software is the same way. Ask the supplier or company representative to furnish you with a demo program or sample screen for trial runs. Be sure demos contain basic commands such as what it takes to add, delete, or update text, graphics, audio, or video files. This is the quickest way to determine if you need programming or if other software tools are necessary. Demonstrations by no means are ironclad guarantees of errorless performance. It just means you've taken healthy precautions before dishing out a bundle of money.

Aptitude for authoring software is not your problem. It's your patience. Using software tools or tools requiring another language at first is an annoyance. But authoring software enthusiasts really boast of the user-friendly instructions and amazing speed of multimedia capacities you can get with sophisticated packages. Table 6.1 provides a preliminary list of product options for you to consider. Jot down which ones sound reasonably feasible given your particular position, personal needs, and budget.

HOW TO SELL YOUR SOFTWARE PROGRAMS

By now, thinking about programming may make you dizzy. You're still skeptical about puzzling commands, help menus, and particularly hidden licensing costs for copying programs. Well, I don't blame you. But authoring software techniques are stepping-stones to more exciting phases of software production—that of marketing. There's nothing more rewarding than observing people apply software you've invented on your computer. When my wife and I created *Rate Your Date,* a survey instrument for mate selection, we sweated bullets that users would not understand our directions and load the software incorrectly. Apparently they did it correctly, or if they haven't, nobody told us.

But I don't think users got the hang of it. Most do-it-yourself programmers create simplified software for users with as little computer expertise as themselves. By reducing technical complexity, users can benefit from your program without the hassles of typing in weird numerical codes or memorizing multiple sequences just to open the program. Keep it easy and keep it fun. One way of knowing if prospective users understand your program is by testing the product ahead of time.

Development and Testing

Introduce your software to a pool of known or unknown users you believe are good candidates for testing. This is unlike forming research groups, where reliability and validity procedures dictate who goes in which group (e.g., control, experimental). Delegating a testing and nontesting group is not necessary. There is no experiment going on here. You're not manipulating independent and dependent variables.

You have only one purpose here: to see if your software works. Groups best suited for software testing include your patients, friends, colleagues, or associates in allied health fields possessing entry-level computer knowledge. You might ask them to load the software following steps on your instruction sheet and see if they could perform a series of functions in the order you specify. Uniformly, have each testing user follow the same sequence as a general measure of consistency. Have your users also test the software on a variety of different computer operating systems (DOS, Mac) and versions of those systems.

Technical glitches discovered along the way instantly help you troubleshoot programming flaws. You can create a working list of common problems, less common problems, and potential problems depending on a user's competency. Questions raised about the program are also important to log. Users may ask why you deliberately left out a specific training step. Well, you didn't; the truth is, you never thought of it. Now you can put it in and save face before hitting the publicity roadshows.

Technical Manuals and Documentation

Ironically, one area mental health practitioners might find easy is documentation. This is the arduous task of describing step-by-step instructions on running the program. You are in effect preparing a *technical manual*. Manuals vary in complexity and dryness. However, writing technical manuals is not terribly different from writing scientific research papers for conference presentations or later for publication. Cautions of writing style apply more in technical manuals than in research reports.

Some writers, for example, overuse jargon for advanced learners who want pointers for accelerated software uses. Other manuals are user-friendly; they realize novice users may consult this text frequently for troubleshooting and thereby leave out excruciating details about basic operations (Dewitt, 1989; Thirlway, 1995; Turk, 1995). You're advised to do the same. For best results, manuals typically contain 11 sections covering application (see Figure 6.1). These include the following:

Installation and Deinstallation

Describe exactly how to get started, from inserting the diskette to copying programs onto the hard drive. A nice touch and frequently available in authoring software tools is to offer an installation program that literally does everything for the user. Now that it's on their computer, be sure to tell users how to get it off their computer. De-installation is a bit more complex than removing the software in

FIGURE 6.1. Sample instruction sheet to accompany software program

Rate Your Date

Installation Instructions

"Rate Your Date" runs best on Windows 3.1 with a mouse. It does not run on DOS, though it can be installed from DOS or Windows.

To install "Rate Your Date" on the computer's hard drive, turn on the computer and let it boot up. Insert the floppy disk for "Rate Your Date" into drive "A" or "B." When this is done, you will either be in "Windows" or at the "C:\>" prompt. Follow these installation steps for either process:

Installing from *Windows*:

Step 1. Your opening screen will likely be the "Program Manager" window, which is the basic "desktop" before you start opening applications. If your computer opens directly into an application, change it so that you are open in the "Program Manager."

Step 2. Read the menu bar under the name "Program Manager." Click on the word "File" with your mouse. Go down the list and click on the word "Run."

Step 3. The "Run" window should open. If you are copying

the floppy disk from drive "A," you must type the following on the "Command Line": **a:\ln stalla.bat**
If you are copying the floppy disk from drive "B," you must type the following on the "Command Line": **b:\install.bat** Click the "OK" button. Then wait for the program to be installed from the floppy disk to your computer's hard drive.

Step 4. Wait until the loading is done and the computer returns to the Windows desktop.

Step 5. To complete the installation, you must click on the word "File" with your mouse. Go down the list and click on the word "Run."

Step 6. The "Run" window is open. If you are copying the floppy disk from drive "A," you must type the following on the "Command Line": **a:\setup.rec** If you are copying the floppy disk from drive "B," you must type the following on the "Command Line": **b:\setup.rec** Click the "OK" button.

Step 7. A new window will open, with "setup.rec" appearing. Double click on the name "setup.rec" to automatically install the program icon onto your computer. Click on the words "setup.rec" again if necessary to start the installation. If this window suddenly minimizes itself (shrinks) and becomes an icon, simply click on this "recorder" icon one time, then click once on the word "maxi-

mize." This should re-open the window with the name "setup.rec." Then start over at the beginning of this step.

Step 8. When the installation is done, a window for a new program group will open on your screen and you will see the icon for "Rate Your Date." Double click the "Rate Your Date" icon to begin the program.

Installing from *DOS*:

Step 1. Your opening screen will likely be the "C:\>" prompt.

Step 2. If you are installing from drive "A" or "B," substitute "A" or "B" as appropriate for your computer:
Type: **A:**
Press: **"Enter" or "Return" key**

Step 3. The screen should show "A:\"
Now type: **installa.bat**
For drive B, type: **installb.bat**
Press: **"Enter" or "Return" key**
Then wait for the program to be installed from the floppy disk to your computer's hard drive.

Step 4. Go to Steps 4 through 8 above ("Installing from Windows"). Follow the installation process as described.

BEST IMPRESSIONS INTERNATIONAL INC.
4211 OKEMOS ROAD SUITE 22
OKEMOS MI 48864
1-800-595-BEST

trashcans (in Macintosh or Windows, for example). Trashcan removals do not actually permanently eradicate products from hard drives. It just makes them invisible. For true hard-drive removals, consider adding a low-cost "eraser" software to your program that works fast and easily.

Quick-Start Steps

Quick Start is a "welcome" screen immediately opening up after the program begins. It outlines in clear, nontechnical language the basic operations and associated keystrokes users need to run the program at its simplest level.

Introductory and Background Materials

Experienced users may skip over this material to some extent, but not entirely. Present a general overview of what your product is, can do, and benefits of its usage. Go on to describe the program's basic operation. A paragraph, or chapter in larger manuals, may offer tutorials guiding users through a series of practice steps. Sample data and templates make tutorials fun and informative. When completed, background information is helpful on advanced applications and interpretation of the user's work. For example, on self-testing personality traits, give users a rudimentary understanding of what these traits are. You double the educational value and chance of users reusing the software or recommending it to their peers.

Main Functions

Present the bulk of how to use the program. List commands, key strokes, or other directly operational tidbits users need in getting through your maze.

Configuration

While optional, frequently users want a blueprint on which way to go and why. Navigation signals on which button to push and when to push it are part of configuration. Discuss available menus and results of selecting options under each menu.

License and Warranty

Basically remind users this product is copyrighted and licensed for personal use, beyond which any commercial application requires your permission in writing (Dratler, 1996). Warranty holds you liable for repair or replacement should faulty programming or other software glitches remain unsolved through telephone support.

Support

Inform users how they can reach you should problems arise. Suggest what they need to describe on-line or by phone for quicker responses.

List of Files and Subdirectories

Lists of new files, or subdirectories of information alert users to updated information and additional tricks, tips, and techniques in case they are adventuresome.

Technical Notes

Questions frequently arise on computer-software compatibility and hardware requirements. Technical notes is an archive for network setup, memory specs, operating system requirements, and other guidelines for interfacing software with other software or other equipment.

Glossary

A glossary is optional but valuable. Consider providing a small dictionary of words used in your documentation. While written in simple English, accidentally a technical word or two can slip in and derail a user's train of thought. Key words defined in a glossary provide fast relief from anxiety, panic, and "Help, I'm a moron" attacks.

Frequently Asked Questions (FAQs)

Complete your manual or one-page description with answers to frequently asked questions (FAQs). Effort spent in advance on troubleshooting means less time spent later in on-line support.

On-Line Help

You may also wish to consider "on-line help." Most programs today incorporate this nifty device to replace boring, over-technical manuals. On-line help either is "menu-driven" or "context-sensitive." Menu-driven helpers appear at the top of the screen and are accessible by pointing the mouse on it and clicking to open it up. An index appears that users may search for key terms they want more information on. Context-sensitive helpers have keystroke magic. When stumbling over a word or character, users just click the mouse button on top of the character or use combination keystrokes. This triggers an automatic display of hints to solve the problem.

SHOULD I MARKET PRODUCTS MYSELF?

Effectively designing a workable software that is user-friendly and fits a niche market is half the battle. Now you can figure out how you want this program to reach potential users. In marketing, several distribution routes exist for product promotion.

Shareware

Shareware is a marketing channel for computer software products and not a type of software. It has one distinct advantage for buyers: they may try the product before buying it and is cheaper than buying it through department stores. Confusion about shareware is common. Many people mistake it for shelfware, public domain software, freeware, bannerware, and demoware. Let's briefly consider what each variation is and how shareware is very different.

Shelfware works through advertisers and requires interested customers to pay first. Shareware, for starters, is free for looking. That's why it's known as *try before you buy.* Shareware is often a smaller working version of the program. It becomes fully "enabled" after the user pays your registration fee and enters a registration number into the program.

Public domain software, by contrast, includes properties for which authors have entirely relinquished intellectual and subsidiary (or secondary) rights. Since 1989, authors must explicitly make that declaration. That also means authors do not collect any licensing dollars for software reproductions or multiple users. Lack of copyright message does not place material automatically in the public domain. Messages are clearly stated by the author. Shareware, by contrast, remains the author's property in spite of offering liberal shopping policies for buyers.

Freeware is similar to public domain in one respect: authors do not demand any payment for specific uses, they reserve their property rights. As in bannerware, a freeware product is a give-away or loss leader in advertising campaigns. Although seemingly free, advertisers pay in advance for software and then in turn piggyback it with new software products. Demoware has the same flagwaving, public relations effect. Examples of demoware are videos, sound waves, and other "working copies" entirely designed as samplers. Picture, for example, "trailers" or movie previews shown on rented videotapes. These video files publicize upcoming video rentals or motion picture releases. As video clips, they are copyrighted and not in public domain. Demoware accomplishes the same goal.

Shareware has many distribution channels. The first is through catalog vendors. Vendors mail their wares to subscribers allowing them to order trial disks from the catalog. A second form is bulletin boards. On-line servers (America Online, Prodigy, Compuserve), including numerous chat and news groups on the internet, make shareware products available for downloading. Users download compressed files through their modems containing both samples of your software and purchasing instructions.

A third way is familiar to you. Office Max, Office Depot, Best Buy, among other national retailers, currently set up racks featuring shareware titles. Shareware even appears on CD-ROM disks. You just select the titles you'd like to try and follow up with payment.

Each of these marketing channels accomplishes the mission of routing your software to buyers. How effective vendors and store owners are at *promoting your software* is a different story. Product exposure may occur slowly, passively, without fanfare, and your software may occupy shelf space for several months. Shareware distributing also has other disadvantages. First, you are not entirely in control over immediate product sales. Trust in the honor system of "use and then pay me" can be unsettling and it may backfire. Downloaded software users may not faithfully pay licensing fees and may simply just "pirate" your brilliant work.

Second, measures of customer profiles and repeat business are hard to track. Reusability of shareware products occurs without your knowledge. Or, if you do know how many programs are out on loan (before payment), details of buyers are unknown. Collecting data on demographics may seem tedious, but it's a lifesaver for targeting a buying market. Where you can, find out who is using your software and for what purpose.

Direct Marketing

For years, direct marketers (DMs) have boasted large sales on products sold through mailing lists. Exclusively compiled lists tailored to your buying population seem a simple and reaffirming system. These lists relieve you of narrowing down customer profiles or searching yourself through infinitely vast bulletin boards in cyberspace, looking for solid matches. Now you don't have to do that. With direct mail, either in snail mail or e-mail, you just rent a list of names or participate in a card deck and wait until purchases file in. In fact, upfront sales produce less profits than revenue from existing customers who pay for upgrades or add-ons.

While a DM method is incredibly easier and offers a true test of your product's viability, some pointers are worth noting on what works and doesn't work in the DM world.

What Works

Here are the types of products that stand a chance in mass mailers. Look at the list below and ask yourself if your product fits into these categories.

1. *Does it appeal to a well-defined audience?* Does your product by its very nature lend itself to a specific group?
2. *Does it have serious retail competition?* If it does, forget it. High-stakes advertisers will probably beat you to the punch with expensive display ads, web pages, and frequent mailers.

3. *Does your product have a moderate price?* Overpriced merchandise belongs in the morgue. Buyers of small software programs usually are thrifty and expect to pay little or nothing for something. Price your product with their garage sale-mentality in mind.

4. *Is your product easily explained?* Self-help software that meets existing needs are best for consumers. Rarely do consumers read details in ad copy. They choose a product based on its name or one-line description under the name.

5. *Is the product perceived as low risk?* Unconditional guarantees help. Customers then know they can return it without questions asked. But "risk" goes beyond that. They want software that is user-friendly, quick to install and perform, and with results that directly benefit their lives.

6. *Will the product result in repeat sales?* Repeat sales in upgrades and product derivatives are better gauges of revenue than initial sales. However, ask yourself if your product is reusable. Can customers work on it every day or discover different results from repeated applications? If yes, that's a strong marketing angle.

Is There More to It Than That?

Direct marketing entails several more steps, such as locating timely and accurate mailing lists (see Ruben, 1995, Chapter 7, pp. 108-110), filing patents and licensing your software, and establishing rapport with catalog sales reps (Schenot, 1995, Chapters 5 and 6). Hard copy versus electronic DM efforts require your time, effort, and expense. There's no way around it. And, even if mailers generate sales leads and produce revenue, expenditures laid out in advance cut into profits. On your labor of love, advertising your software through some DM channels may barely recover your costs.

Selling Electronically on the Internet

Have I destroyed your software ambitions? I hope not. Recall that, for books and magazines, electronic communication by far was a stronger way to reach your party. Electronically selling software products is not any different. For instance, take the internet. Merchandising on the internet is big. Industry leaders quote Cybersource Corporation's success. This manufacturer grossed over $10 million last year from 400 to 500 orders per day across some 8,000 software products advertised on-line. Of those products, 70 were electronically downloaded, with more being added monthly. Because electronic distribution largely eliminates packaging costs and distributor, guess who benefits? The buyer. Significant savings can be passed along in lower pricing. To date, Cybersource is the only software distributor on the web providing this value-added service.

How does Cybersource pull this coup on the web? Here's how. It's back to shareware. Offer prospective buyers an evaluation of the product to download for free. If they like the product, they're invited to send money to you or your company. But here's the best part: Since users with web access typically work for large companies, you, the software manufacturer, can telemarket into a location where a number of copies have been sold and sell the user's companies a site license.

Advertising on the internet is like a 24-hour continuous trade show. Attendees at the show exist on varying mailing lists you can access from databases online. Lists are in abundant supply *if you know where to look and if you use a little creativity to leverage different websites.* Why buy a list of, say, 5,000 names costing you $500 to $1,000 when you can go into cyberspace for free? You can currently go to various free websites and download as many basic data files as you want within minutes.

Some sites are intended for job seekers. They may carry as many as 10,000 companies in their databases; other lists are shorter. The size is up to you. Simply enter a search engine such as Yahoo and type in key words describing your target group. For instance, type in "anxiety" if hoping to generate website lists and chat groups of patients or therapists treating anxiety. Lists you compile can be privately and selectively downloaded, or copied and pasted onto a word processor for a later database. Within literally seconds, you'll be rewarded with your own buyer sample ready for software testing.

Beyond company mailing lists are a host of speciality weblists. These feature e-mails and a litany of people-finder resources. They are easy to use, fast to download, and perfect for merchandising. Round up lost relatives, high school classmates, and subject-specific groups such as volcanologists, college students, and international internet users. All peculiar subgroups are accessible at the click of our legless mouse. Table 6.2 contains a sampling of such sites you should definitely check out.

TABLE 6.2. Sample of specialty weblists

American Directory Assistance
http://www.abii.com/lookupusa/adp/peopsrch.htm
Contents: Provides up-to-date phone numbers for people nationwide.

American Universities
http://www.clas.ufl.edu/CLAS/american-universities.html
Contents: A directory of college and university home pages. Use to find a school, and then search for students and employees.

Bigfoot
http://www.bigfoot.com/
Contents: An e-mail directory that boasts 4 million entries and claims to grow at a rate of one million new entries every month.

Classmates Online
http://www.classmates.com/
Contents: Find your old high school alumni. More than 15,000 schools are registered here.

Four11 White Page Directory
http://www.Four11.com/
Contents: More than 6.5 million listings of e-mail addresses and phone numbers.

Internet Address Finder
http://www.iaf.net/
Contents: Almost 4 million e-mail addresses are listed here.

Switchboard
http://www.switchboard.com/
Contents: A whopping directory of more than 90 million names and phone numbers.

Volcanologists List
http://www.aist.go.jp/GSJ/-jdehn/vnews/vlist1.htm
Contents: Largest list of volcanologists reachable through internet.

World E-Mail Directory
http://www.worldemail.com/
Contents: A directory with an international flavor that lets you search by continent; boasts more than 9 million entries.

Federal Trade Commission (FTC) Rules

The good news is that you can legally take shortcuts reducing your outlay of costs and late-night hours spent on marketing. Now for the not-so-good-news: Not every trick is legal. Soliciting orders and receiving payment of any sort through snail mail and e-mail falls under rules of the Federal Trade Commission (FTC). This organization sets standards for marketers assuring ethical and fair business practices. Rules pertaining to software sales comprise their "Mail Order Rules." Essentially, these rules require that direct marketers operate according to the following rules:

1. Do not advertise something that you cannot ship within 30 days of the order.
2. Clearly and conspicuously show your order processing time or that orders can be processed within 30 days.
3. Clock the time on order processing from receipt of a completed order to delivery of a properly addressed package to the shipper.
4. Provide an "option notice" if you cannot ship the product in time. This means notifying customer of shipping delays and offering an option to cancel the order.
5. Provide a detailed explanation for the delay in the event you cannot give a specific shipping date.
6. Provide in writing to customers action you will take if customers don't respond, such as stating that a nonresponse signifies cancellation of the order.
7. Provide a "renewed option" letter to customers if notification of an "option notice" (#6) is null and void. A nonresponse from customers on renewed option letters is an automatic cancellation of the order.
8. Provide a complete and prompt refund if you cancel the order. Refunds must be sent by U.S. first-class mail within a week of the cancellation.
9. Ship exactly what customers ordered, particularly on option notices.
10. Guard against overuse of the word "free." Orders received for a "free trial period," for example, cannot require payment. However, one slight change gives you leverage. That is

if you include a bill-me-later option as well as a way for customers to send money.

Federal rules governing the sales trade are fairly strict and may only supplement state or county rules. A safe business practice is calling your local or state Chamber of Commerce for clarification of rules and any updates immediately affecting your sales activities.

AUTHOR'S CORNER

Below is a summary of questionnaire replies from software authors who kindly shared their insights, frustrations, technical information, and tips for beginning authors.

Summary of Replies from Sample Software Writers in Mental Health and Allied Fields

1. **Background and degrees:** BAs in computer programming, psychology; MAs in computer programming, experimental psychology; no PhDs
2. **Number of software programs sold:** 2 to15
3. **Number of software programs written but not sold:** 10 to 25; areas include mailing databases, word processing, games, interface and Novell networks, astrology, nutrition, personality surveys
4. **Number of technical manuals sold:** 2 to 10 (with or without software sold)
5. **Lag time between submission and acceptance:** 1 to 3 months
6. **Lag time between acceptance and production:** 4 to 8 months
7. **Range of advance received upon acceptance:** $250 to $1,000
8. **Range of royalty percentage received (on retail, wholesale) or outright purchase price:** outright price is $2,500 to $5,000; royalty on retail is 5 percent to 8 percent
9. **Tips offered to newcomers in software writing/development:**

   a. Be creative with your ideas after you've spent time playing with software.

    b. Find a programmer who you can collaborate with.

    c. Stick to your specialty area. Ideas come faster, and technically you're smarter.

    d. Get more jobs as technical writers for documentation. Few computer operators know how to write well. They would hire mental health researchers over data technicians for writing manuals.

    e. Look at what's selling fast. Don't duplicate it, but borrow from its graphic technology on creating your own product.

RESOURCES

Walk into any software store from Software City and CompUSA to Best Buy. Look up and down the aisles of education, graphics, and business software products. It's like a beehive. Getting dizzy? I would. It's so confusing that, thank goodness, salespeople twice and three times younger than you can find out what you need in seconds. How disheartening, though, when they report the software you want is out of stock, or better still, is obsolete. You feel like a dinosaur. Been out of touch with new products and progress in computer hardware?

Big mistake. As you already knew and this book reminded you, good software sells quickly and then it's gone–forever. There's no such thing as a "golden oldie" of software. System upgrades, internet access upgrades, and software upgrades all fuel the velocity of the computer industry speedway.

As one company's software corners the marketplace, another company's product disappears into oblivion. The raging fury of software companies to pass one another in the regatta is hard to keep up with. It's like nobody wins; companies just take turns in the lead. That is why many companies listed in Chapter 9 may have successful or unsuccessful products by the time this book is published. However, listed companies all share one denominator in common: they sell both smaller and larger software products, licensed with larger corporations and smaller business owners. They spread out in their sales and service fields.

All the entries are open for original software submissions. Contact a small number of companies at first until you feel comfortable.

Your best shot, as explained earlier, is to be brief. That is why only fax numbers appear in the entries.

REFERENCES

Dewitt, H.S. (1989). *Secrets of successful writing: Inside tips from a writing expert.* New York: Reference Software International.

Dratler, J. (1976). *Licensing of intellectual property.* New York: Law Journals Seminar-Press.

Ruben, D.H. (1995). *Publicity for mental health clinicians: Using TV, radio, and print media to enhance your public image.* Binghamton, NY: The Haworth Press, Inc.

Schenot, B. (1995). *How to sell your software.* New York: John Wiley & Sons.

Thirlway, M. (1995). *Writing software manuals: A practical guide.* Englewood Cliffs, NJ: Prentice-Hall.

Turk, C.C. (1995). *Writing effective software documentation.* New York: Routledge, Chapman & Hall, Inc.

Chapter 7

Industrial and Infomercial
TV Producers

Not too long ago, my wife Marilyn teased me about writing too many academic books. She said I really needed a career change. So, I listened to her. She described this funny idea of writing movies—not just for glamorous motion pictures but all types: TV shows, commercials, and infomercials. We even spent a "second-honeymoon" at Northwestern University attending Richard Walter's one-day scriptwriter's workshop. There I got a glimpse of tinseltown's finest scribes and heard insider tips on breaking into showbiz's most underrated profession: screenwriting. Still curious and at my wife's urging, I wrote a screenplay and sent it out to producers in the wild blue yonder.

Well, we haven't sold that screenplay yet. But diving headfirst into scriptwriting later opened doors of opportunity for educational scripts and infomercial scripts to TV pilot scripts. Can you enjoy a similar transition and keep your 9-to-5 mental health job? Yes, I believe so. That's what this chapter attempts to show you.

Here's what it won't show you. It won't inflate your hopes of selling a million-dollar screenplay. While aspiring scriptwriters can follow this dream and pitch their screenplays, I advise you to take the low road first. Dealmakers are always on the prowl for literary properties with high box-office sales potential. But why shoot for the stars when you can reach the clouds faster? Writing for corporate videos and infomercials earns you faster experience in the ropes of the trade (Abreu and Smith, 1996).

In no time, you can understand do's and don'ts of scriptwriting and speak videoese. Confidence in your writing expands the challenge to teleplays or pitching new TV shows, whether documentaries, sitcoms, or educational programs. Exciting avenues you take depend as much on writing fervor as on boldly asserting yourself in unfamiliar territory.

Is it always unfamiliar? Will there be a time when writing, pitching, and negotiating deals in TV business will seem second nature? Probably, but not for a while. Even industry experts can't feel at home. They discourage complacency. They realize that between silicon valley techno-changes and roller-coaster dealmaking, yesterday's rules are today's exceptions (Froug, 1993; Kosberg, 1991; Litwak, 1994; Stuart, 1994).

Be awake, they advise; purge old beliefs and jump onto Hollywood's fastest treadmill in reaching producers. This reflects a major change in Hollywood politics. Harvard MBA agents using "Wall Street" tactics are faster, smarter, and trash old rules for negotiations. They're bulls in a china shop and have created twice as much work for scriptwriters, but at great expense. Egos bruised and profits gouged, today's producers are doing their own recruitment; they use fewer literary and casting agents. The trend has caught on. Scriptwriters and actors alike are representing themselves and finding stable employment. Higher wages, longer contracts, and versatile work comprise the entrepreneurial commerce of freelance scriptwriting.

With opportunities expanding, you have a choice. You can either wait on the street corner or take the next subway into your dreams. Go with your gut feelings of doing what hundreds of practitioners discovered is possible. Stimulate your writing growth to astonishing rates in only months. Check into scriptwriting as an avocation and see where it gets you. Are you ready? Okay, read on, and see how it works.

WHAT'S HOT, WHAT'S NOT

Fiscally minded producers will tell you up front: if it doesn't grab the public by the throat, it's no good. Why do sitcoms such as *Married with Children, Ellen, Seinfeld, Home Improvement,* and *Murphy Brown* reappear year after year? They're hilarious. Contract renewals for 20 to 30 episodes means job stability for staff writers, producers, and other above-the-line and below-the-line workers. Shows scoring big in Nielson ratings are picked up by national affiliates (CBS, NBC, ABC) and run for years because advertisers want to sponsor them and because viewers remain loyal.

TV show winners frequently are in comedy, but a good crime or hospital-based drama can equally steal the Peoples' Choice awards. Triumphs of *Chicago Hope, E.R., Homicide, Law and Order,* and *NYPD Blue* all reflect efforts to feed viewers watered-down realism short of repulsion. Even shows depicting graphic violence, such as *Cops, Emergency 911, Real Stories of the Highway Patrol,* and *L.A. Firefighters* teeter on repulsion but soften the harsh blow with moralist commentaries.

Shows enjoying success on TV are recycled versions of big-screen attractions. Unequivocally selling more tickets are comedies and hard-core crime stories. Recently, *Cable Guy, The Nutty Professor,* and *Father of the Bride Part II* grossed multimillions in their first weekend releases. Thrill-seeking, special-effects spectaculars such as *Eraser, Independence Day,* and *Mission Impossible* shoot high-voltage excitement into white-collar murder and mayhem. Audiences crave this torturous collision course between crime, fate, and human frailty. Villains, heroes, and bystanders build story suspense, are hugely popular, and draw whopping box office numbers. It amounts to a simple formula: adversity in movies is the prime ingredient for megahits.

With these TV shows and movies influencing adults and children, all other shows expected to turn a buck must follow the crowd. Infomercials, documentaries, and educational or corporate videos priming for a buying market, in some way must interplay with viewer taste. Below are the hottest trends in these particular markets and how they borrow from large-budget prototypes in the industry.

Interactive Education and Videoconferencing

Supersonic transmissions of voice, video, and graphics from your monitor to monitors thousands of miles away is rocking the computer industry. It replaces telephones, video sales, and cellular phones. Even beepers are getting a run for their money. Software downloaded from internet bulletin boards makes it now possible for simultaneous communication between large groups of people. The buzzword is *videoconferencing*. Videoconferencing really isn't that new. Ten years ago, Fortune 500 companies tested videoconferencing for jet-set business travelers attending meetings in foreign countries. Video relays were slow and sound quality deteriorated in static, but overall connections were made. The idea? For one face to see another face over the computer.

Educational videos teaching step-by-step use of videoconferencing and internet-friendly competency are in demand. Instructionally showing which software to use, how to operate systems, and tips against mechanical glitches round out a perfect scenario. The trouble is that videoconferencing still has limited markets. Corporations already employing this technology are begging producers for updated teaching films. Smaller firms, even those networked worldwide, may feel investing in desktop videocameras for face-to-face dialogue is wasteful. Instead, they'll putter along in DOS or Windows 3.0 until linking computers in other countries simply cannot "talk" to them anymore.

Writing scripts on videoconferencing requires an obvious background in computers and a creative layout for scenes. For example, training can revolve around a story of two videoconferencing businesspeople, both cashing in a company deal. Or, tailor videoconferencing to employees with families who can maintain visual contact with loved ones while out of town.

Comedy

Corporate scribers are notorious for using comedy (DiaZazzo, 1992). Flippant jokes, humorous vignettes, and off-beat storylines bolster viewer enjoyment and rapidly get the message across. Monty Python alumnist John Cleese appears in many industrial films parodying employer interviews, coping with difficult people, and sexual harassment on the job. His inimitable style as straightman plays off unsuspecting actors who fall into his hilarious traps. Cleese's ingenious comic videos top the leading training video rentals and purchases to corporate buyers.

Cleese, like his competitors, realize that the funnybone has a direct line to memory. Information presented in comedy training films is retained longer and inspires subsequent workplace changes. So, too, infomercial scripters are joining the comic bandwagon by selecting celebrity comediennes as product spokespersons (Cooper, 1994).

Docudrama

Film festivals worldwide from Cannes to San Francisco's Outfest are showcases for independent movie producers. They display their wares in front of critics and peers prior to widespread theatrical release. Festivals also test out shark-infested waters of agents, distributors, and actors sneering at competition but open to picture deals.

Sure, they look at Steven Spielberg's colossal productions. But they also look for artistic and documentary films. Dramas inspired by realistic events that deeply changed the lives of a family or company are popular. These are called "docudramas." Dramas entirely based on facts and unfolding incredible tales of human victory, defeat, survival, and torture are purebred documentaries.

Whether a documentary or docudrama, teleplays in this genre receive attention. And here's why: as 500+ cable channels hit the airways, many carried over far-reaching cable systems such as TCI, programming needs for each channel will grow. Channels ambitiously expect to fill 24 hours of programming. Some will actually accomplish this goal, especially those sponsored by larger networks. Privately owned channels such as the *Children's Cable Network* and *Arts and Antique Network* (see Chapter 9) may struggle filling their programming slots. They will auction slots to independent producers who have series proposals or have completed pilots and episodes and are looking for TV exposure. Other producers wishing for a piece of cable action may not have writers on board or a ready portfolio of pilot shows. They openly welcome solicitations from new writers on pilot ideas fit for cable or network channels.

Business and Management

Innovative products for human resource development and managing one's own personal growth fill the video catalogs for today's trainers. Industrial videos singularly address one question: How can I motivate employee performance? Their answer: by graphically presenting vignettes, animations, and instructional videos on leadership, organization, creativity, conflict resolution, time management, and even insider tips on giving training seminars. Each video is a mini virtual reality engaging viewers to pretend they are facing actual tough work problems. Frustrations that viewers identify with in work situations are demonstrated by the video's protagonist, who then experiences a series of lessons. We see a trainer enter the picture, giving advice on the protagonist's problems, or the video may shift to a purely educational format. Following this learning segment, we return to the protagonist, who now applies his or her new skills under frustrating situations.

Secrets of effective video presentation lay in capturing honest and accurate employee obstacles. Recently, for example, videos offered advice in response to downsizing, layoffs, cultural diversity in the workforce, providing accommodations under the American Disabilities Act, and guidelines for averting sexual harassment. Whether used as part of large-group training or watched individually, videos are essential helping tools for everyday work adjustment.

For starters, pick up a recent video catalog from a video company and peruse their listings. Fit your idea into their selections, modifying this with your creative improvements or insights on real-life employee or employer obstacles you hear about in clinical sessions. For example, "documenting discipline" is a phrase included in many video titles. But suppose your clients report repercussions in intraoffice politics when favorite, yet bad, employees come under fire. Your spinoff idea for this video, then, combines "discipline" methods with strategic diversions for "office politics." You'll be surprised how interested producers will be, especially since your ideas derive from their target buyers.

Vanity, Greed, Power, Success, Love

Educational and even infomercial videos long have been copycats of basic human impulses: vanity, greed, power, success, and love. High-powered, product-pushing videos, for example, on kitchen appliances, are not boring. They addictively lure viewers into a feeling that this product is indispensable for their daily cooking needs. Compelling messages almost seem subliminal. Underneath the barrage of fast-talking sales pitches and dazzling video graphics were neurally programmed commands to buy the product. That's because producers knew what grabbed gullible viewers: anything that viewers valued as essential to their lives. Products, story lines, or characters obsessed with physical attraction, making money, accelerating success, enhancing romance, and jumpstarting careers up executive ladders all fill this human void.

Lately, another strong human passion is tempting video producers: action/adventure. A morbid taste for violence comes from blockbuster thrill-seeking movies such as *Judge Dredd, Terminator, Terminator 2, The Fugitive, Terminal Velocity, True Lies,* and a host of others (Troy, 1996). Viewers live on a compulsive diet of seeing people graphically terminated. They endure nail-biting tension between heroes and villains, waiting impatiently for somebody to pull the trigger, and outsmart and outperform the enemy. As special effects wizards ingeniously find new ways to satisfy this craving, action/adventure genres with less technical genius are also popular.

Your goal in scribing an educational or commercial video is not to duplicate Hollywood entertainment. It is, though, to jack up the action or suspense in some context in order to *grab* viewer interest and generate believable reasons for buying products or listening to advice.

SCRIPTWRITING 101

How well can you convey your ideas in scripts? Do you rigidly follow rules guiding plot development and product description, or is your style more extemporaneous? Is it better to be spontaneous than overkill on details? Which style is better for organizing sequences and product promotion? Scriptdoctoring gurus have mixed opinions. One camp of L.A. experts definitely advise a military regimen. They advocate conforming to a specific number of pages, certain plot twists, and a two- or three-act format unless writing educational videos (Ballon, 1992; Davis, 1994; Reichman, 1992; Segar, 1992; Segar and Whitmore, 1994; Trottier, 1995). On the Beverly Hills side are advocates of the creative process. Experts may suggest some roadmaps but largely encourage using your imagination; they stress writing freedom and paying more attention to hooks, action, and dialogue (Walter, 1988; Wolff and Cox, 1991).

Whichever approach you take, be sure of one thing—your net result *must look in some way like other scripts in the industry.* In Chapters 11 and 12 in *Publicity for Mental Health Clinicians* (Ruben, 1996), I provided examples of technical scripts, teleplays, and even scripts for motion pictures. Rather than duplicate this material here, consider this an update. Industry-changing trends and new software will keep your scripting current and ahead of competition.

Industrial Scripts

Technically different in educational and industrial scripting are the multimedia formats. With CD-ROM and interactive video markets rising, producers want scriptwriters who are skilled in the arts and crafts of audiovisual graphics. Line your page with two columns. Title one column "Video" and the other column "Audio." List under the video column action scenes involving animation or real-time people interaction. Under the audio column, list corresponding dialogue, music or other sound selections. Dialogue may be between two people seen on the screen or without action, as a voiceover accompanying, for example, graphic displays. Voiceovers provide the sound while the viewer watches figures, tables, a series of instructions, or montage of pictures, people, or other rapidly shown video clips.

Script lengths will vary, but stick with the standard of 15 to 30 pages, with each page being one minute long. Training videos beyond 30 minutes are exceptions, as, for example, in high-profile promotional pieces supplementing product presentations or as part of a larger advertisement campaign. In such cases, videos may be adapted for cable or network TV.

The guaranteed way to ensure your format conforms with industry standards is to play it safe: Contact producers ahead of time and ask for them to fax you a page from one of their recent scripts. Notice if your layout contains key words and follows a similar sequential order of scenes. By matching your script to this prototype, instantly your script is compatible with the producer's expectations and enhances your credibility in writing experience.

Infomercial Scripts

Writing for infomercials–now called "Direct Response TV"–has undergone revolutionary changes. Ten years ago, a handful of infomercial producers led the pack with million-dollar returns on high turnover products. Sales writing was an in-house staff job, usually done by producer acting as director, acting as scriptwriter. Combining jobs saved on overhead expenses and allowed for bigger spending on TV airtime slots. Now, with direct response TV cashing in faster on many products, and through endless outlets, such as infomercial channels and home shopping networks, demand for freelance writers is greater.

Hired writers currently receive not only a writing fee but are enjoying "points." Points are back-end fees or percentages based on the show's product success. Up-front fees of $5,000 to $18,000 plus expenses may be paid against projections of $10,000 to $50,000, depending on whether writers negotiate for 5 percent or a higher cut of net profits. Your percentage of net profits constitutes your "points."

Payoff of points is not as nebulous in direct response TV as it is in motion pictures. Accounting practices in larger productions can hide, divide, and eliminate proof of net earnings or in fact show grave losses, thereby delaying back-end payments to investors. But dollars earned on infomercials operate on a simpler accounting system. You can track the paper trail between buyer orders, product fulfillments, labor and production costs, and even staff and postage costs. In all, monitoring expenditures versus income is procedurally easier and more reliable. That is why more celebrity spokespersons, producers, writers, and product inventors are willing to accept small salaries in exchange for higher percentages of profit.

Today's infomercials have glitz, shine, and polish. They run a tight time frame of 28 to 30 minutes of demonstration, live audience, testimonials, and spots. "Spots" run anywhere from one to three minutes and look like commercial breaks. In effect, they are breaks, but of a certain type. They are stop-segments for viewers to know how to order the product. The 800 phone number, costs, and purchase options such as monthly payments and use of credit cards are given. Spots occur three times during the infomercial: one at about 8 to 10 minutes, another at around 20 minutes, and the third one at end of the show. Spots fit into several current formats, including live audience, demonstration and magic, story and testimonials, news and talk show, and celebrity pitches.

Live Audience

Live audiences are recruited by promotion or production companies. They consist of previous users of the product, potential users, or just a random gathering of friends and families. Audiences are carefully coached to respond enthusiastically at specific times. Arousing claps and cheers generates a feeling of spontaneity, authenticity, and is *exciting* to viewers who can identify with audience reaction.

Demonstration and Magic

Literally write in a segment where the spokesperson or inventor displays the product. Use the strength of TV media to get watchers salivating at how effectively the slicer-dicer, juice machine, cosmetics, or hypnotic stop-smoking tapes really work.

Story and Testimonials

Identify previous happy customers willing to share their experiences. One-on-one interviews disclose not only their deep satisfaction with the product, but radical changes it made in their lives. In one infomercial, individuals sang the praises of hypnotist Damon Reinbold for eliminating their three-pack-a-day habit of 30 years and preventing risks of cancer. Testimonials laudably boosting the product, product inventor, and touching the sentiments of millions of watchers are incredibly powerful. Best of all, satisfied customers are usually eager to share their success stories. Where stories tell of miracles, testimonials are more than powerful; they lock in sales.

News and Talk Show

Initially, infomercials borrowed the concept of the talk-show format for selling products. Today, the format follows an "Oprah" type of show or "Letterman" behind-the-desk style. Spokespersons act as TV hosts, introducing segments of the show and visiting the studio audience. Intersperse this format with personal, one-on-one interviews with previous product users. A twist on this theme is a news-anchor structure; here, one or two newspeople (preferably a man and woman) sit behind a table reporting on the product as if it was a late-breaking story. Reporters "on the scene" provide updates and in-person interviews with the product inventor or spokesperson. The entire segment resembles any local newscast.

Celebrity Pitches

For shows promoting brand awareness or product image, celebrity spokespersons are perfect for making pitches. This makes the product more recognizable. Celebrities add glamor to products and heighten viewer interest if the spokesperson is known in TV or movie circles. Watch the ecstatic buyer reaction when, for example, heartthrob Dylan Neal of *The Bold and the Beautiful* displays his physique alongside a pair of hydro-knives. The telephone lines would heat up! Hydro-knives would sell at astonishing rates.

Keep in mind celebrity figures when outlining your infomercial topic. As you structure segments, consider some other common elements. Direct response TV scripts typically follow eight steps. While not carved in stone, these steps ensure your script incorporates effective strategies for merchandising power. Include in your format an introduction, problem-solving pitch, hard-sell message, the spot, the promise, education, running tease, and testimonials.

Introduction

At the beginning of the show, establish your host, establish the show's format, and target your audience by identifying the problem you are going to solve. For example, describe a heavyweight show-host mixing in the live studio audience, announcing that "Today on Amazing Inventions, watch as smokers become nonsmokers, once and for all."

Problem-Solving Pitch

Remember that your goal is to sell a product. One way of compelling viewers to pick up the phone and place an order is to show how the product solves a problem. Have the spokesperson, celebrity guest, or inventor pose multiple problems and explain how this miracle product is the answer!

Hard-Sell Message

Push comes to shove just before a spot or commercial-like break. The host appeals to the buyers' basic human needs (greed, vanity, fear, fun, laziness, etc.) with an arousing, evangelical pitch. "You'll never find anything like this . . . never!" Ironclad guarantees convince shoppers the risk is low and benefits are enormous. *Hey, why not? It's not that much money.* That's right, just dial that 800 number and ring the ever-buzzing cash register, raking in profits.

The Spot

Write in a two-minute summary of the show's product and value it has for consumers, plus details on how they can purchase it.

The Promise

Promises are more than money-back guarantees. Hosts, previous users of the product, and the inventor give honest reassurances of how you can be happier once this product is in your life. Validate their claims by having users say they never wanted to return the product.

Education

Background is vital but don't overkill on education. Explain essentially why the product works in lay language, using simple-to-understand points of science. Refer, for example, to research, but water it down to a sprinkle and highlight only relevant results. "A study conducted on 100 smokers showed that hypnosis eliminated the habit faster than traditional therapy and without side effects." Now, that statement is commanding.

A little edification using experts also goes a long way. On two infomercials, for example, I served as a "psychologist expert" endorsing a particular product to treat addictive habits. Thirty seconds of my "I highly recommend product X for its fast relief of misery and addiction" and audiences are convinced. Why? Because *authority speaks the truth.* Honest professionals who support your product or tried it themselves are perfect candidates for endorsement.

Running Tease

Vaudeville pitchmen were sensational at the running tease. They'd open a show alluding to a fantastic feat to be described later and would stretch buyer interest as long as they could before exposing the feat. News anchors on your local news station do this regularly. They frequently flash clippings of a big story to hook you into viewing weather, sports, and local news until two minutes are left in the broadcast. That's when the big story is covered. By then, you've seen all 30 minutes of news.

Testimonials

Testimonials seem simple but are reportedly the most difficult components of infomercials. Previous product users share personal, compassionate stories on how your product incredibly changed their lives. Solid, credible testimonials not only are fast product sellers, they also show Mr. and Mrs. Average in normal predicaments (e.g., needing help, cash-poor, watching TV), discovering super-normal happiness. Late-night and early-morning viewers vicariously can identify with Mr. and Mrs. Average and decide what's good for those happy campers is good for them.

SCRIPTWRITING SOFTWARE

Organizing your thoughts in direct response TV or other commercial video writing is easier when you have software telling you what to do. Think of it as your personal writing companion. Scriptwriting software available for Mac and IBM has been updated since I originally reported on them in Chapter 11 of *Publicity for Mental Health Practitioners* (Ruben, 1996). Today's upgrades feature lightening-speed interactive tools, a dictionary, thesaurus, and even on-line creative help files guiding plot development. For computer neophytes, there is user-friendly software with fewer keystrokes and operating similar to normal word-processor programs. On slightly more complex levels, features include script formatting, story analysis, outlining, and character building.

Scripting software usually accelerates the creative process. But before you test-drive a program, ask yourself these questions:

1. How easy is it to learn?
2. How well does it allow me to make changes?
3. How well does it implement different script formats (film, infomercial, audio-video, etc.)?
4. How easy is it to transfer files to and from other programs?
5. How comprehensive is the support provided by the vendor?

The bottom line is this: convenience in writing is a matter of processing speed and uninterrupted flow of typing. Spooner's (1996) comprehensive review of screenwriting software considered these points. She voted *Scriptware* the best overall program on the market today. It is easy to learn, allows creative juices to flow freely, and can interface with standard word processing software. Table 7.1 lists other variously priced scripting software to consider.

TABLE 7.1. Scriptwriting software programs

Software	Requires	Price	Contact
Collaborator II	Mac/Power PC Windows	$330	Collaborator Systems 800-241-2655 800-405-8344 collaborator@msn.com
Dramatica-Pro	Windows Windows 95	$299.95	Screenplays Systems Inc. 800-84-STORY
Final Draft	Mac/Power PC Windows	$350	B.C. Software, Inc. 800-231-4055 www.bcsoftware.com/ bchome OR info@bcsoftware.com
Moviemaster	Windows 95	$234	Movie Master 201-251-1979 mmsupport@aol.com
ScriptThing	Windows Windows 95	$199	ScriptPerfection Enterprises 800-450-9450 KenSchafer @aol.com
Scriptools	Windows Windows 95	$99	800-4647511 72154.1251@ compuserve Mac/Power PC
Scriptware*	DOS, Widows	$299.95	Cinovation, Incorporated 800-788-7090 http://scriptware.com
Side by Side	Windows Windows 95 Mac/Power PC	$79.95	888-234-6789 SimonSkill@aol.com
Writing Screenplays	Mac/Power PC DOS	$39.00	Macro Concepts 310-459-2195

*Note: Scriptware is voted best overall program for novice and seasoned scriptwriters.

REFERENCES

Abreu, C. and Smith, H.J. (1996). *Opening the doors to Hollywood: How to sell your idea-story-book-screenplay.* Los Angeles, CA: Curtos Morum Publishers.

Ballon, R. (1992). *Blueprint for writing.* Los Angeles, CA: Write Word Press.

Cooper, J. (1994). Lights, camera, profits? Infomercials clogged with celebs. *Broadcasting and Cable, 124(3),* 80.

Davis, W. L. (1994). *Screenplay companies: A workbook for screenwriters.* Carson, CA: A Write-Side Productions Book.

DiaZazzo, R. (1992). *Corporate scriptwriting: A professional guide.* New York: Focal Press.

Froug, W. (1993). *The screenwriter looks at the screenwriter.* New York: Silman-James Press.

Kosberg, R. (1991). *How to sell your ideas to Hollywood.* New York: HarperCollins.

Litwak, M. (1994). *Dealmaking in film and television industry: From negotiations to final contracts.* Los Angeles, CA: Silman-James Press.

Reichman, R. (1992). *Formatting your screenplay.* New York: Paragon House.

Ruben, D.H. (1996). *Publicity for mental health clinicians: Using TV, radio, and print media to enhance your public image.* Binghamton, NY: The Haworth Press, Inc.

Seger, L. (1992). *The art of adaptation: Turning fact and fiction into film.* New York: Henry Holt & Company.

Seger, L. and Whetmore, E.J. (1994). *From script to screen: Collaborative art of filmmaking.* New York: Henry Holt & Company.

Spooner, E. (1996). The ultimate screenwriting software review. *The Journal of the Writer's Guild of America, 9,* 24-38.

Stuart, L. (1994). *Getting your script through the Hollywood maze.* Los Angeles, CA: Acrobat Books.

Trottier, D. (1995). *The screenwriter's bible.* Los Angeles, CA: Screenwriting Center.

Troy, P. (1996). Lethal weapons: Action/adventure writers. *The Journal of the Writer's Guild of America, 9,* 14-18.

Walter, R. (1988). *Screenwriting: The art, craft, and business of film and television writing.* New York: New American Library.

Wolff, J. and Cox, K. (1991). *Successful scriptwriting.* Cincinnati, OH: Writer's Digest Books.

Chapter 8

Wake Me Up from Dreamland:
Hard Truths of Selling Scripts

Scriptwriting can take a monetary toll on your wallet if you are not careful. Hidden costs for software, agents, expert opinion, attendance at workshops, and shipping scripts out for review all click away at the dollar meter. Still, is it worth it? I think so.

Calculated planning on what you write and who you write for may save you time and effort. Decide which genre is comfortable for you. Educational and corporate scripting? Infomercial scripting? The choice is yours. But in thinking your direction, realize that scriptwriting is not an open writer's market. Rivals are everywhere. Would-be scriptwriters from zero to 30 years of experience compete for a premium parking space in congested lots. Even veteran writers are not safe. There is no such thing as scriptwriter's tenure. You are never "vested," but rather "tested" by each and every property submitted for review. No one person is secured a contract.

While fighting through crowds to be noticed, figure that your odds of a big break are greater because of two facts. First, you have intuitive wisdom as mental health experts able to write on human behavior. Second, you'll be equipped and ready to handle any calamity. The worst disaster, of course, is facing rejection. Let's talk about rejection for a moment. Then, I'll share some tips on how to undermine competition when selling corporate and infomercial scripts.

UGLY REALITIES OF REJECTION

Have you ever gone through emotional peaks and valleys? At one moment, ecstatic, and hours later, mellowed out like a couch potato? Cyclical mood swings are the culprit. Scriptwriters vying for a piece of showbiz struggle with mood swings. They soar into aerospace when hearing their script is liked and under review; nothing else matters. Totally absorbed by unlimited possibilities, they picture themselves in a new career, doing what they love, and being paid royally for it.

Then it hits like a ton of bricks: rejection. The "Dear John" letter politely refuses your script, adding good wishes to your ventures elsewhere. But by then you feel disillusioned and start questioning your motives for scriptwriting.

When you embark on the do-it-yourself venture of selling your scripts, rejection is unavoidable. True, you wrote the script hoping to sell it. You may also have found it therapeutic and lots of fun. Still, dollar signs were going off as you packaged and mailed it off to producers. How many dollars? Several.

If you were planning on making a million dollars, forget it. Chances are that it won't happen—not right away. That's the reality of the scriptwriting business. Other ugly realities plaguing the submission process are valuable to know so you can prevent cyclical mood swings and pragmatically strategize solutions to your disappointments.

Most Scripts Do Not Sell

Scripts for commercial, industrial, or direct response TV stand a better chance than TV and motion picture scripts, but most scripts submitted over the transom do not get picked up. The script that sells is usually your second or third attempt rather than your first one. One or two scripts let you experiment with the craft of writing, and frequently mental health providers pick up quickly on format and rhythm. But winning instant prize money for a first-time script option is unlikely unless your topic is incredibly newsworthy or you've collaborated with an established writer.

Most Scripts Are Optioned, Not Sold

Scripts acquired by producers are done on an "option" basis. This means producers want to reserve rights to your script while they raise funds for a production. Options are for three months to one year, depending on projected budgets. Payment for options varies considerably. Producers may try asking for your script for free, but otherwise pay from $1,000 to $5,000. If funds are not raised in time, rights revert to the writer.

Most Scripts Optioned or Sold Are Not Produced

Scripts passing the screen test of being optioned or even sold outright still run aground. They may never be produced. Even seasoned, successful scriptwriters in business and TV industry have many scripts never put before cameras.

Most Decision Makers Are Young

This point may be irrelevant for many readers but deeply fearful for still other readers. Many executives given decision-making roles in the video and film industry are between ages 20 and 35. By 35 years old, they either rose to higher executive branches or formed their own production company and oversee general operations. Underlinks in charge of creative development, acquisitions, and programming are fresh out of college and many are not even writers themselves. They rapidly inherited overwhelming responsibilities learned "on-the-job" (Kulakow, 1996).

A way around ageism is not to advertise your age or use extensive metaphors or case illustrations alluding to the 1940s, 1950s, and 1960s. For example, leave out of the dialogue references to *Gilligan's Island* or *The Lone Ranger.* While these classics may be appreciated by viewers of the video, producers and directors who make the video may not have the foggiest idea what these shows are.

Most Out-of-Towners Struggle at First

Fear abounds that residents outside of Orange County have no chance of breaking into the scriptwriting industry. True, you may have a more difficult time getting a networked agent. True, travel and correspondence may be awkward and limit appearing in person. Nonresidents are only at a disadvantage if they put all of their eggs in L.A. baskets.

What about the other 49 states? Michigan, Florida, and East Coast headquarters for infomercial and commercial producers lately have stretched Hollywood boulevard across the nation. Florida, in particular, threatens to be the next movie capital with Universal, MGM, Paramount, and several independents soaking up the Atlantic coastline. So, keep a global eye on the buying market to expand your prospects.

HOW TO RATE YOUR INFOMERCIAL PRODUCT IDEA BEFORE IT AIRS

If you think about it, the idea really is revolting. Had you mentioned to somebody 10 to 15 years ago that millions of people would be willing to sit down in front of their television at an ungodly time of night, watch a commercial, and then order some product by phone–wouldn't that person have thought you were crazy? Probably. But not anymore.

In the last ten years, long-format television commercials have generated an astonishing billion-dollar-plus marketing industry. And it hasn't slowed up. It's gaining momentum at warp speed. Infomercial savants such as Guthy-Renker and William Sergio took average products, paired them with recognized faces (e.g., Micky Rooney, William Schallet, Lyle Waggoner, Steve Allen, Linda Gray, Dick Gregory, Bill Bixby), cashed in on commercials disguised as entertainment, and it worked. Five million dollars a year in sales were recorded since 1984, when the government ended its 12-minute-per-hour limit on TV ads.

Now infomercials or direct response TV, are part of mainstream television. The trouble is that with hundreds of commercials airing, viewers are growing more particular with their tastes. The public knows what's good and bad. They can spot a piece of junk and turn off the channel in seconds. Generating high sales volume requires shows that are creative, sensitive, and persuasive. That's why writers attuned to consumer behavior are precious gemstones to producers. Insight on buying trends and how to push the right buttons for sales is all the marketing they really need.

One bit of insight you can help producers with is making the infomercial more believable. Your writing may incorporate convincing elements, from testimonials to hard sell. But are there other ways to rate the show before it hits the broadcast airwaves?

Yes. Here are reliable yardsticks of product success to keep in mind while writing initial copy or rewriting drafts:

1. Have you written in a loss-leader product to generate immediate responses? Loss leaders are giveaway products that entice the buyer to want the premium product. Giveaways may be books or accessories such as a set of knives, all delivered "free" if the buyer purchases the meat defroster for $95.99.
2. Never invent a product from scratch. Eligible infomercial products are already moneymakers. Proven success is important because TV is a mass medium and proven appeal weighs heavily on success. Consider that every household that turns on the TV is a potential buyer. Does the product appeal to widespread groups or only upscale or niche markets, that is, a very small percentage of the viewing market?
3. Select and exemplify a product that has demonstration power. Let it cause a magical transformation right before the viewer's eyes. Car polishes, kitchen gadgets, even height phobics walking up ladders fit this category. When you can show a problem and introduce your product to provide a solution to the problem, you've got a crown winner.
4. Select a product that truly solves a real problem. Products such as weight-loss programs and smoke stoppers hit home with habit-trapped viewers. They sink massive dollars into quick-fix cures if they see a light at the end of the tunnel. But they can't conclude the product helps if it is a preventive measure. Insurance benefits, for example, never sell. The same goes with bratbusting strategies for busy parents who need help managing unruly kids. Unless the kid is a terrific nuisance wreaking havoc for everyone, it won't sell.
5. Introduce a back-end or "upsell" potential with your product. "Upsell" means you want to get the buyer on a continuity program or develop your business for reorders. Vitamins for sexual enhancement, for example, require refills. Work it into the script that mail-order refills may earn dollars toward a yearly vitamin magazine subscription.

How to Target Infomercial Audiences

Making an infomercial is a costly venture. Shows cost from $100,000 to $500,000 and testing how well the infomercial sells directly to TV viewers will run from $30,000 to $40,000. To test retail sales impact, producers run the show ten times in sample regions of the country rather than exploding it nationwide. Depending on the size of sampling markets, airtime costs can average $20,000 to $50,000 per market. That is why, as writers, you want a solid lead on who your market is.

Over the past years, infomercials chased stay-home moms and late nighters. But now, adult viewers are second to the $95 billion teen market. Many teens watch up to four hours of TV daily. The nation's youth may be naive shoppers, but their gullibility invites an infomercial bonanza. Marketers are creating snappy, 30-minute TV commercials that look like MTV shows complete with rock music, loose language, and young stars. Forget that adolescents don't have credit cards. Commercials tell teens where they can call for information on buying the products. For example, sled dogs, the $329 in-line skates for snow, are in a commercial about a dog chasing a teenage boy. Spots lasting a few minutes urge young buyers (ages 13 to 20) to purchase the product.

Whether videogames or minidisks, teen-targeted infomercials represent a capitalizing market. Can other populations be targeted for a commercial you plan to write? Sure there are. For example, early-bird TV viewers include the 60+ seniors. Entice this demographic group with panaceas for persistent medical ailments limiting happiness. Cures for psoriasis, impotence, memory lapses, and even creams guaranteed to wash away aging wrinkles will sell big.

One series of 15-minute and 30-minute infomercials stressed safety; a life-saving device worn around the neck acted like a "garage-door opener." When activating it, electrically transmitted signals triggered your telephone to dial 911 for a medical emergency—no fuss, no family, no go-betweens. Elderly disabled consumers seized this product to gain control of their lives—a fantastic steppingstone to independence.

The same has been true for successful infomercials on retirement programs. M & T Bank's 30-minute show "The Power of Annuities" described the benefits of tax-deferred annuities. First-run markets aired only in New York State, specifically Albany, Syracuse, Rochester, Buffalo, and Westchester County. Viewers were offered the opportunity to request more information and an application kit by dialing an 800 number. Other financial institutions taking a similar infomercial plunge are Fidelity and American Express.

Some targeted audiences are easy marks. Other targets slip into gray areas requiring a clearer definition of who they are and what you want from them. Select your best TV audience based on consumer buying habits of the product you want to sell. Consider, for example, the following:

1. What is the monthly average consumer purchasing of your product?
2. What is the sales volume of similar products advertised on TV?
3. What is the viewer *acceptance ratio* of your product? "Acceptance ratio" is involved in two variables. The first is the believability of product information delivered by everyday types of people (testimonials) and credible experts. The second is their product identification. This is when your show creates a personal sharing experience between viewer and spokespersons. Minutes into the show you want the viewer to say, "Gee, I have that situation too." If they do, your product hits the dollar bullseye.
4. What volume of services does your target audience seek for relief of some problem cured by your product? Physician appointments, therapies, bookstores–wherever they go–may rank top priority in their frustrating daily routines. You want your product to solve their miseries faster and more efficiently.

Why Infomercials Fail

Offering a product with integrity and solutions captivates viewers, but it may not be enough. It is estimated that over 250 to 300 infomercials are currently on the air around the clock, clogging up cable and broadcast television. Thirty to 60 new infomercials appear every month from sunrise to sunset. With the 500-channel universe just about open, lower advertising rates will lure multichannel runs for longer periods, suffocating the airwaves even more. In effect, paid direct response TV is verging on epidemic proportions from a writer's standpoint, thank you. You have a lucky break. Capitalize on vast opportunities to enter inside the "sacred corridors." But, infomercial critics are less enthusiastic: they warn writers that hooking up with a "sounds like a moneymaker" show can turn sour if serious mistakes are made in the early stages.

Even the best-laid plans of mice and men backfire when five unforeseen errors creep into infomercial planning stages. Be aware of these suicide traps now before you put too much time into the project:

1. *Never sell a regular product just on its laurels.* Marketing directors mistakenly believe they can sell their standard product based on its research or past sales record. They assemble a simple commercial pushing their product with little or no punch, thinking consumers already know how good the product is. The trouble is that infomercials are not purely silent billboards. They talk, act, and carry more messages than a dictionary. Be sure the marketers realize consumer awareness means *information plus satisfying personal needs.*

2. *Never overdo the entertainment.* Some dreamy-eyed marketing director may budget for a Busby-Berkeley-like musical extravaganza. He figures splashy entertainment filled with streamers, firecrackers, and big-name celebrities is a sure bet. Remind him, however, that while infomercials should be fascinating, *the purpose is marketing, not entertainment.* His goal is to sell, not get ratings. The mistake is this: they spend 24 minutes with bopping heads or sitcom format or glitzy entertainers, and throw in three two-minute product commercials.

   Don't do it. You'll miss the mark. Instead, be a chemist. Blend the ingredients of showmanship with hard-sell product information.

3. *Don't sell more than one product in your infomercial.* Multiple product sales confuse consumers and sound as if you're padding the offer to make a quick buck. One product is plenty for a 30-minute show.

4. *On risky products, lower the budget.* Spending more doesn't guarantee high sales projections. On moderately tested products or products enjoying success through other media (e.g.,

mail campaign), keep costs reasonable and below the average $250,000 to $500,000. Better the talent be a familiar face than a blockbuster, and format of the show be subdued to simpler, less expensive segments.

5. *Hire big guns to do the job for you.* One type of rejection letter you'll receive might say, "Gee, we're sorry; only hiring seasoned pros. Try again in ten years" When this happens, figure this infomercial will die. Caliber of expertise of course is important in directors, talent, and most below-the-line staff. But infomercials are not a rocket science, and creative decisions for what effectively whets consumer appetites will not be obtained from traditional scriptwriters or media-buying agencies experienced purely in retail product advertising. Input from hands-on experts is mandatory and that is where you always fit in. It's okay to remind decision makers of this. Let them know you have an irreplaceable role.

REPRESENT ME FOR A PRICE?

Publicity for Mental Health Clinicians (Ruben, 1996) described in several chapters the advantages and disadvantages of using agents to represent your work. In scriptwriting, agents certainly have a louder voice if they truly interface with industry movers and shakers in infomercials, and educational and industrial videos. What follows is an update on why agents should be treated as the late actor Orson Wells eloquently said about wines, *We'll sell no wine before its time.* With agents, I'd advise, *They'll sell no play until you pay.*

Pros and Cons of an Agent

Getting an agent is challenging under the best of circumstances. Getting the best agent for free or little money is even a more daunting task. It just doesn't happen. When it does—when neophyte writers get signed by an agent—writers are so thrilled they fail to ask the right questions early in negotiations. "Costs?" you later ask yourself, "I thought they only worked for their ten percent." Well, not really. They earn ten percent later on and a host of fees up front or pretty near to up front.

Representation simply is not a free ride. After signing, plan on sending four, five, even up to ten copies of your script. That means you'll be paying for copies and postage. And that's only the beginning. Writer's Guild of America (WGA) signatories may not be able to charge reading fees, but watch out for clerical and processing services running up the meter before your script is sold. Phone calls, written correspondence, even reimbursement for luncheons or meetings with prospective script buyers may be billed to you.

One enterprising agent made it easier for his clients. He charged a flat quarterly fee of $75.00 for overhead costs. Clients naturally presumed this $75.00 went toward promoting their scripts, and maybe some of it did. But with 50 clients, all paying $75.00 four times a year, he's assured a guaranteed income of $15,000. Sure, it's not enough money to buy a yacht, but it's plenty for possibly doing absolutely nothing. So, watch out: *You'd be paying into the agency welfare system.*

Unscrupulous agents are like the Phantom of the Opera. The mask they wear hides a hideously greedy face. While writing this chapter, for example, I received an industrial script rejection urging me to contact an editing firm called *EditInk.* Call it a coincidence. I heard from other writers who received rejection letters from other companies also referring them to *EditInk.* While none of these writers objected to professional editing, they all were curious why *EditInk* figured so prominently.

I don't know why, but I do know kickbacks occur frequently between agents and editing firms. *EditInk* or another editing firm may charge you $5.00 per page and rebate the referral source $1.00 per page. Fees for summaries and critiques can run into the thousands. That's hundreds of dollars commissioned back to the referring source. Scams built on a pyramid of commissions outsmart you by cultivating your fantasies of million-dollar script deals. One script consultant's pitch went this way: "(We have) created a series of reports on the screenplays and pitches that were sold in 1995 and in the first quarter of 1996!" Other editors lay it on the line with an outright punch of reality:

> I don't know how happy or unhappy you might be with what I tell you about your script or book, but I promise

you this: what I say or write to you will be constructive and sincere, based on knowledge, not this week's hip and jargon and hype, and will bring with it 20 years of experience as a screen and television writer and producer.

However eloquently they word it, gullibility is what they're after. Temptation to use their services instead of personally struggling with newcomer mistakes is your fatal mistake. Even your clinical acuity doesn't spot this trap in advance. That is why selecting agents or adjunct editorial services is a matter of careful shopping. Before you bite the bait, carefully investigate editors for hire including research on their past clients and book projects. If they are agents, ask about their success at placing manuscripts and scripts with publishers and producers.

PROPOSING NEW TV SHOWS

Writers are quick learners. After working remotely or in house for several productions, you rapidly pick up on the routine and process. Who to hire, which equipment to rent, where to get cast and crew insurance, location and talent contracts, scheduling, and most important, how to talk in *entertainmentese*. For example, "get a *grip* on it," doesn't refer to facing reality. It means asking a staff person called a *grip* to handle cameras, lights, or other equipment paraphernalia. Speaking the language is as important as knowing something else: Can your commercial video undertaking materialize with a reasonable budget and with you behind the helm? Do you have what it takes to become director, producer, editor, and writer all at once? Sure you do. You just need to know how to do it.

In the last ten years, with fewer studio giants, one-time employees of large studios have formed their own *independent companies*. Independents represent a major revolution in the entertainment industry for two reasons. First, independents make their own administrative, budgetary, and talent decisions rather than slaving to studio executives. Second, ancillary services such as lending institutions, insurance agents, print and advertising, publicity firms, talent agencies, and domestic and international film distributors openly invite relationships with small production firms. This allows underdogs to compete on equal footing with giants such as MGM, Orion, Paramount, Warner Brothers, Universal Studios, and Disney, among others.

Many innovative producers who originally operated on shoe-string budgets making popcorn (B-rated) movies evolved into prime time and box office heavyweights. David Kelley Productions (*LA Law, Chicago Hope, Picket Fences, Mixed Nuts, The Practice*), Witt-Thomas Productions (*Brotherly Love, John Larroquette Show*), Aaron Spelling Television (*Beverly Hills 90210, Melrose Place, Savannah, Seventh Heaven*), Ten Thirteen Productions (*X-Files, Dark Skies*), Miramax (*The Postman, Jane Eyre*), New Line Cinema (*Ninja Turtles, Rumble in the Bronx*), Gramercy (*Fargo, Cold Comfort Farm*) all freshman production companies, soared into million-dollar stratospheres following repeat hits.

What got them started and continued their momentum was doing everything *their own way.* And you can do it too. Self-producing, like self-publishing, thrives on personal endeavor. While aggravating and unspeakably complicated at first, once you get the bugs out of the system and follow a routine from start to finish, you'll wonder why you didn't begin your scripting career this way.

Being Your Own Producer

Picture this scenario: You've just seen CNN report on the early morning bomb blast in Atlanta's Centennial Park, killing two people and injuring 100. This overshadows Olympic festivities and once again reinforces terrorism destroying ideals of peace and brotherhood. You're struck with the genius idea of a 30-minute talk show exploring similar tragedies, trauma, and even the supernatural. So, immediately you flip through your local TV guide, perusing for any current shows resembling your concept. Good, none so far. Now you write a summary featuring key points of the TV show and any host you believe has local, regional, or national celebrity appeal (e.g., see Figure 8.1).

That was easy. You've completed the first step of independently producing a commercial video or TV show. You identified a concept in writing. One-page synopses for variety talk shows, situation comedies (sitcoms) (see Figures 8.2 and 8.3), and documentaries are exactly the same. Describe in simple words the basic plot or

FIGURE 8.1. Synopsis for a video or TV show

Exploring the Psychic
with Joyce Hagelthorn

Produced by
Best Impressions International Inc.

4211 OKEMOS ROAD, SUITE 22, OKEMOS, MICHIGAN 48864, U.S.A.
TELEPHONE or FAX: 517-347-0944, or 24 hrs at 517-347-1811: 1-800-595-BEST

Show Summary

TALK SHOW ON SUPERNATURAL

Local celebrity star and former editor of Dearborn Press, Joyce Hagelthorn has dazzled the airwaves for eight years with her spectacular, high-rated talk show on the psychic and supernatural. *Exploring the Psychic with Joyce Hagelthorn* is a one-hour show, taped live in front of a studio audience and run weekly on both Cablevision and Continental Vision. Hundreds of prominent guests from Dr. Marcello Truzzi, International expert on debunking ghosts, to Dr. Charles Lietzau, national biologist and explorer of crop circles, join a host of psychics with incredible feats. Nowhere on TV is there such probing inquiry on UFOs, paranormal, and hidden dimensions confronted in a lively, entertaining style. Call-in questions make *Exploring the Psychic* a powerful interactive TV show, filled with compelling facts, figures, and fantastic phenomena.

Host Joyce Hagelthorn is no newcomer to paranormal study. Over 20 years ago, she began writing her weekly column *"I Never Told You But ...Exploring the Hidden Dimensions of Natural Events"* (Media Press, Nebraska). She also pioneered the *Do Something Different* training seminars hailed as Michigan's outstanding patron series. Joyce's debut in TV with *Exploring* propelled her popularity overnight, with Cablevision subscriptions significantly increasing. Four years later, Continental Vision picked up her show, asking her to do a second live show from their studios.

Exploring the Psychic with Joyce Hagelthorn uniquely stands alone in talk shows with high-energy excitement mixed with a calming brew of informative education.

FIGURE 8.2. Synopsis for a variety talk show

Celebrity Talk Show
with Michael Dante™

Produced by
Best Impressions International Inc.

4211 OKEMOS ROAD, SUITE 22, OKEMOS, MICHIGAN 48864, U.S.A.
TELEPHONE or FAX: 517-347-0944, or 24 hrs at 517-347-1811: 1-800-595-BEST

Show Summary

Celebrity star Michael Dante, who has appeared in over 30 motion pictures, 150 television shows, and spent seven years under contract with MGM, Warner Brothers, and Twentieth Century Fox, has been radio host the last three years of *The Michael Dante Celebrity Talk Show*, live on KPSL, Palm Springs, direct from the Marriott Desert Springs Resort and Spa. His half-hour variety show features such famous Hollywood guests as Tony Curtis, Milton Berle, Sidney Poitier, Jerry Vale, Frankie Avalon, Buddy Hackett, Larry Gelbart, and such megasports stars as Johnny Bench and Don Drysdale. Now this playground of the stars comes to television in **The Celebrity Talk Show with Michael Dante.**

This half-hour entertainment show presents the latest inside scoop on a celebrity's activities, from obstacles to ovations felt from Tinseltown to Broadway. Dante's unique debonair grace unravels amazing true stories from his guests. Since most of L.A.'s best are his personal friends, high-profile stars of over three decades, loved by millions of viewers, regularly appear on his show.

Dante's exciting career started as a major league baseball player, rapidly evolving into starring roles in *Winterhawk, Cage, Beyond Evil, Willard, Arizona Raiders, Return from The River Kwai, Westbound, Kid Galahad,* among several others. His recurrent roles in sitcoms and daytime soaps made him a household name, appearing in *Cagney & Lacey, The Trials of Rosie O'Neill, Knot's Landing, Days of Our Lives, Simon and Simon, Star Trek, General Hospital,* and *The Insiders.* Over 100 additional episodic roles round out his continuing streak of acting in motion pictures and TV guest spots. Michael also commuted to Dallas, TX for several years to host the half-hour variety show *Dallas Alive.*

Demo audiotape available from radio show.

FIGURE 8.3. Synopsis for a situation comedy

WHAT'S COOK'N?
A Best Impressions International Inc. production
in association with Patton Barry Productions

4211 OKEMOS ROAD, SUITE 22, OKEMOS, MICHIGAN 48864, U.S.A.
TELEPHONE or FAX: 517-347-0944, or 24 hrs at 517-347-1811: 1-800-595-BEST

Title: What's Cook'n?

Length: 30 minutes

Frequency: Once weekly.

Producers: Best Impressions International Inc., Patton Barry Productions
Executive Producers: Doug Ruben, Alyce Faye
Writers: Doug Ruben, Alyce Faye, Marilyn Ruben
Music: Doug Ruben

Purpose: In the spirit of *Home Improvement* and *The Larry Sanders Show* comes an irresistible new sitcom featuring Motor City comedienne Alyce Faye as "Alyson the Chef." Together with her quivering cohost, Philip, **What's Cook'n** is a weekly food show that goes every which way but right. On the air, Alyson's sharp wit pumps guests for the "food obsession" they must have, while she cynically fingers Philip's endless goof-ups, hang-ups, and flops. The compulsive type, Alyson is a walking and talking food machine who taste-tests the food Philip makes. Of course, wimpy Phil's smiles and dry jokes suck up to his big boss Alyson's willingness to keep him on the show and let him bunk at her apartment. Offstage, friction erupts between producer Saperfeld's "everything-for-a-buck" mentality and Alyson's unlimited appetite for food and "got-to-have-it-match" demands. If the drapes don't match because they cost too much, that's one Saperfeld-Alyson boxing match you don't want to miss on HBO. On the lighter side is Alyson's miserable love life coming off as Annie Oakley the gunslinger scaring off every sweet guy she finds. Nothing like her blond and beautiful, guy-catching best friend Samantha (Sam). She draws guys like flies, but loses them overnight. And while Alyson tries to clean up her act, Philip keeps pampering her wounds and Saperfield wonders if the network was drunk when they hired Alyson.

Live Audience: None, but laugh track

Proposed episodes: Pilot plus one episode taped in local studio under production staff of (tentatively) September Moon Productions

Format: 30-minute show with three commercial breaks lasting 120 minutes each. Each commercial break has estimate of four commercials at 30 seconds each.

format, followed by publicity hype for the host, celebrity star, or projected marketing impact on certain viewers.

Accompany the synopsis with a brief inquiry letter (see Figure 8.4). Letters follow a simple format of four paragraphs. First, present the angle and reasons for writing. Second, introduce yourself as producer of a dynamite show and add glowing descriptors that help embellish the plot, host, or anything relevant to the proposed show. Third, promoting a host means singing his or her praises in high pitch. Do a musical number on the star's showbiz history, including a round of "celebrity geography." Indicate celebrities the host knows, has worked with, or is best friends with. Finally, remind the cable or network company what you want—to be in their programming schedule. A list of possible prospects appear in Chapter 9.

Producing on a small scale—the best way to get started—involves two more steps. The first is *fiscal priorities*. The second is *maximizing your personal resources*. Fiscally prepare yourself for a home-grown project. Budgets of 30 million, similar to techno thrillers *Waterworld* or *Jurassic Park,* are unrealistic. Think small, think simple. Be a prudent accountant. Start with a budget under 500 dollars, paying for as little equipment purchases, rental, or staff as possible. Low budgets keep your creative juices flowing since you end up doing most of the work yourself. Construct a ledger or list to create a good understanding of your tasks. This list assigns line items with projected necessary expenditures, including scriptwriting, site, equipment, wardrobe, talent, and miscellaneous items incurred during preproduction, production, and postproduction (for extensive production reports) (Honthaner, 1993). The following is an example of a list you might draft:

Preproduction

1. Location site fees	$50
2. Music needle-drop fees	$50
3. Scriptwriting	$0
4. Equipment rental	$100

Production

1. Talent (host, interviewer)	$100
2. Music needle-drop fees	$50

Postproduction

1. Editing and duplications	$100
	———
TOTAL:	$450

Controlling costs means you creatively find ways to rally exist-ing resources in your grasp that can be used for free. *Maximizing your personal resources* essentially is where you either secure equipment or services for gratis, barter, or deferred payments. In the chart above, notice how ridiculously low fees appear for film loca-tion sites, talent, equipment rental, editing, and scriptwriting. Here is why: either you can do the work yourself (e.g., scriptwriting) or hire jobs based on a clever swop between services and benefits. Paying the talent $100, for example, falls well below minimum Screen Actors Guild (SAG) union scales for even low-budget shows, but can act as up-front money against later or "deferred" interest in the show. Back-end interest is called "points." A percent-age (2 percent, 5 percent, 10 percent) of gross or net earnings from selling the show either by direct marketing or by cable/network licensing agreements can compensate the talent.

Deferments reduce initial overhead, especially when you already know where the show will air and how much money you expect to make from it. When future revenues are not known, deferments are still possible as long as some product merchandising related to your project can show earning potential. For example, retail sales on books, audiotapes, and T-shirts about the show can be counted on to pay deferment points.

Vendors of services (equipment rental, film location site fee) are also strongly receptive to *barter* arrangements. Barter is when the service they provide either gratis or dirt-cheap gets them a deal; in turn, they receive a comparable service from your end. Location site is a good example. Near me, for example, there is a historic village consisting of relocated, preserved homes from the late 1800s and

FIGURE 8.4. Inquiry letter to accompany synopsis of TV show

BEST IMPRESSIONS INTERNATIONAL INCORPORATED

4211 OKEMOS ROAD, SUITE 22, OKEMOS, MICHIGAN 48864, U.S.A.
FAX or PHONE: 517-347-0944; PHONE: 1-800-595-BEST; local 347-1811

Mr. Tom Mazza   January 23, 1995
Senior Programming Vice President
PARAMOUNT NETWORK TV
5555 Melrose Avenue
Los Angeles, CA 90038-3197

Dear Mr. Mazza:

Our production company represents several investors strongly encouraged by cable and TV programming and who desire to back new projects featuring celebrity entertainment. That's why we're interested in the *PARAMOUNT NETWORK TV.*

Best Impressions International Inc. is a Midwest teleproductions firm that puts together pilot shows for new and established cable and TV channels. Our most recent is *Celebrity Golf Show* for The Sports Channel. But for the *PARAMOUNT NETWORK TV,* we have a powerhouse show in mind. We'd like to produce a talk show pilot featuring Palm Springs' hottest personality—radio, TV, and movie veteran Michael Dante. Dante has hosted a weekly radio celebrity show live from the Marriott Desert Springs Resort and Spa. On cable or TV, it will become **The Celebrity Talk Show with Michael Dante.**

Dante's guest list reads like a "Who's Who" of Hollywood, with regulars Milton Berle, Sidney Poitier, Jerry Vale, Frankie Avalon, Buddy Hackett, Larry Gelbart, and megasports stars Johnny Bench and Don Drysdale, among others. This one-hour variety entertainment show filmed in Palm Springs gets an insider's look on what's happening with the stars as they start new projects. It's a behind-the-scenes peek at talent from acting, directing, and producing sides of the camera.

Enclosed for your initial review is a show summary. I would be happy to discuss this pilot further with you and to see how we can add **The Celebrity Talk Show with Michael Dante** to your outstanding schedule of programs.

I look forward to your call.

Very sincerely,

Douglas Ruben
President
Best Impressions International Inc.

early 1900s. Exteriors and interiors are ideal for period shots in dream sequences or for historical documentaries. I arranged to pay them a small filming site fee in exchange for widely publicizing their village. Other vendors may barter for opportunities to be in front of the camera or continued use of their services. Talent, for example, may agree to a lower up-front fee if they can secure a spot in subsequent episodes of your show.

Ingeniously negotiating with vendors for barter or deferment can help you keep your costs down and under control. Still, there are fixed costs (e.g., needle-drop for music licensing rights) and hidden fees typically stretching the budget at the last minute. Hidden fees include food, transportation, makeup, and wardrobe. Think about it. Somebody has to feed the two or three cast members during a shoot. A "BYOF" (bring your own food) deal simply won't fly. Transportation to and from shooting sites can accumulate mileage expenses not only for yourself but for each cast or crew member. On-camera talent may need a professional makeup artist for special light-deflective treatment, unless the talent can apply his or her makeup, which they frequently can.

Hidden costs are not saboteurs to your under-$500 movie budget. They simply inflate projected figures more or less depending on your dealmaking integrity, flexibility of vendors, and talent you work with.

Raising Money for a Show

Of course, filmmakers will argue that the best way to finance commercial movies or videos is to use other people's money (Litwak, 1994; Wiese, 1992). Up-front loans borrowed from trusted individuals called "investors" is a tricky business and requires clear definition of what the money is used for and payback schedules. Investors are venture capitalists seeking opportunities for aggressive return on their dollars. Sure, they can prudently invest in mutual stocks paying 8 percent to 10 percent interest over a two-year period and ride out market fluctuations until they cash in. But they are not that conservative. Venture capitalists are risk takers without being irresponsible gamblers. They are open to 10 percent to 15 percent return rates on sizeable contributions of anywhere from $5,000 to $50,000 (on very low-budget projects) where the waiting period for payback and profits is short (six months to one year) and nearly guaranteed.

"Nearly guaranteed" does not mean an absolute deal. It just means you cleverly obtained prelicensing agreements with a cable channel or buyer for sales upon delivering the film. Those earned dollars promise not only recovery of investor's loans but also payment of profits. Investors enjoying 40 percent of net revenue, for example, would recoup their loan plus receive additional hundreds or thousands of dollars simply for sticking their necks out.

Figure 8.5 presents an investor proposal fact sheet for *The Celebrity Talk Show with Michael Dante* (see also Figure 8.2). Notice the total projected budget is $30,000. Inquiring investors are requested between $5,000 and $10,000 up front. In return they stood to earn 40 percent of the producer's net profits. Net profits are the amount of dollars remaining after all expenses are paid. Forty percent assures the investors get a huge piece of the profit pie. Pie-splitting, however, can be more generous. Higher budgets require higher payoffs, considering the risks involved; pay investors 50 percent to 60 percent of the profits. While shrinking your own take, be mindful that whatever you earn is entirely due to charitable backers. You are their beneficiary and remain constantly in their debt; in other words, *never be mean, greedy, or evasive to investors, and never bite the hand that feeds you.*

Do's and Don'ts of Investor-Backed Productions

Finance-backed productions provide several advantages for you. First, you take less financial risks with your own money, except for some preproduction or advanced costs simply to get the ball rolling. Preparing and copying proposal documents, calling friends, talent agencies, and location sites–each of these incur minor costs. Second, investors give your show *prima facie* credibility. You instantly have the clout to effectively speak in entertainment language to vendors, talent, and crew. The language, you ask? Money. *Money talks.* Promises based on expectant finances are a dime a dozen. Promises backed up by solid investor-committed funds supporting your production opens the right doors. You can coordinate the entire above-the-line and below-the-line jobs without ever

FIGURE 8.5. Investor proposal fact sheet for proposed TV show

Celebrity Talk Show
with Michael Dante™

Produced by
Best Impressions International Inc.

4211 OKEMOS ROAD, SUITE 22, OKEMOS, MICHIGAN 48864, U.S.A.
TELEPHONE or FAX: 517-347-0944, or 24 hrs at 517-347-1811: 1-800-595-BEST

FACT SHEET

How much investment money is needed? $30,000

How much do you need to invest? $5,000 to $10,000

What percentage of profit is paid to investors? Forty percent of the producer's net profits (after all production costs paid for the pilot show)

When is your investment paid back? Initial investment is paid back immediately after the show sells. Sales are to cable networks, to national networks, or to other stations (network/independent) who buy the show. Payment of profits occurs after all production costs are paid. On the pilot, profits are distributed after initial investment is returned and after covering any other outstanding production debt in the budget.

How much does that earn you on your investment? You will receive your initial investment back, plus a percentage based on the number of investors and how much they invest. The following is a breakdown showing returns for four investors:

	Investment	Percentage	If net profit is $10,000, 40% of it = $4,000
Investor 1	$5,000	15%	$600 (per show) x 6 episodes
Investor 2	$5,000	15%	$600 (per show) x 6 episodes
Investor 3	$10,000	35%	$1,400 (per show) x 6 episodes
Investor 4	$10,000	35%	$1,400 (per show) x 6 episodes

Who is the check or money order made out to? Best Impressions International Inc.

Where is the money deposited? In Dean Witter Account, East Lansing, Michigan

Who uses the money and how is it used? Executive Producer, Doug Ruben of Best Impressions International Inc., will use money to pay all vendors (services) for the pilot production.

Are there any perks? Yes. Investors whose shares are $10,000 or above will enjoy an expense-paid trip to Palm Springs to watch the filming.

receiving a penny if dealmakers witness signed documents proving your "money is where your mouth is."

While miles ahead of nonfinanced shows, investor deals pose several problems that are best to approach from the outset. First, profit-sharing for investors is only viable if there are profits. Shows not generating revenue either to recover loans or pay dividends are a bust deal for investors. Contracts that entirely bind the investors just to profits, not ownership of the show, leave investors without any real legal recourse to reclaim their money. For example, if investors sign a contract promising them payback of their loan plus points *if the show earns profits,* and if profits are not earned, investors lose their money and may have to walk away empty-handed.

Of course, venture capitalists rarely get into such snags. They prevent financial disaster by forming a corporation. Called a *limited partnership,* investors collaborate to pay a certain dollar amount as the extent of their liability. Partners act as shareholders of this corporation, the purpose of which is to produce a video, TV, or commercial film. Money loaned defines the shareholder's stake in the claim. How much a shareholder contributes is equal to how many shares he or she owns in the company. If one investor contributes $50,000 to a $100,000 budget, that investor owns 50 percent of corporation stock.

Limited partnership corporations serve one valuable purpose: they protect investors against default. Stockholders are monitors policing all stages of production, including expenditures, timetables, and fulfillment of licensing deals either for merchandising, cable channel slots, or, in some cases, theatrical distribution. Watchdogs of invested capital not only are the stockholders but elected officers of the corporation who have the freedom to hire independent accountants, attorneys, or other experts to verify operations are going smoothly. Problems are dealt with immediately instead of reported later; the money chest is vaulted against unscrupulous action.

Still, problems may occur. Shows can be filmed, edited, and delivered to their cable locations following precise steps outlined in the limited partnership. Although the producer has kept his or her word thus far, making money at commercial video or movies is less automatic and cannot be an ironclad guarantee. Shows that do not earn money and appear headed toward bankruptcy have one last shred of hope for investors. As stockholders, they hold title to assets of the company. Assets consist of several things, such as (a) rights to the name of the show, (b) the show itself, and (c) any legally binding contract for licensing rights. A majority stockholder who is an investor can fire the producer, paying him for his services or buying out his or her share if the producer also is a stockholder. With the producer gone, investors can hire another producer and reedit the show to resuscitate it.

Efforts to protect the invested money never are perfect. Even legally binding partnerships have loopholes where producer may wiggle out of stockholder's strongarm. Upsetting the apple cart, as you might imagine, destroys the trust and honesty investors had in a producer, and further reflects negatively on the entertainment industry. One sure way of mitigating problems with investors—whether investors are your family, friends, associates, or independents—is to hire an entertainment attorney. Let this expert draw up tightly knit partnership agreements. Your goal is to make a product, not be your own legal counsel. A solid contract with investors proves you are credible, professional, honest, and, frankly, a good risk.

Making Your Own Video

Since Edison's kaleidoscope days, it has been traditional for the producer to be his or her own cinematographer. Shoot your own film, direct your own script, and hide in your own editorial pod during postproduction. It's an accelerated trip in visual storytelling. Struggling directors and producers without investor funding find do-it-yourself videos an innovative alternative to failure. Self-made videos are popular for production demonstration, industrial training, and low-budget talk shows (Hampe, 1993; Morley, 1992).

Product demonstration videos (promos) usually highlight one particular product and include specific information, such as what the product looks like, how it works, the cost, and how to purchase it. Promos are often viewed at expos, conventions, and retail stores so passersby will stop, watch, and buy the product.

Training videos specifically educate employees on new applications, policies, or equipment. In fact, once the training session is on tape, there's less pressure to hire a speaker or facilitator. Still, home-made training videos also can be sold as adjuncts to workshops and seminars.

TV shows use do-it-yourself videos to allow for ease and flexibility in shooting schedules, location sites, sets, and changeover in camera operators. You can avoid hassles of union pay scales, congested shooting schedules and multiple layers of grips, camera, and sound personnel by limiting your staff to yourself and possibly one or two other people. For example, my wife Marilyn assisted me with scripting and filming a documentary news show on tracing family roots. She displayed the choreographed action while I operated the camera and directed the scene. We used our children to show adults as children in flashback segments.

"So, fine," you say. "I pick up a Sharp video camcorder, wireless microphone system, and that makes me Cecil B. Demille?" No, it doesn't.

But here's what does. How do you turn amateur hour into professional videography? Go back to computer basics. Did you ever notice that your local TV news uses bullet charts and video interviews in split-screen windows? MTV, king of graphics, runs videos at a deliberately low speed to imitate a high-tech look. Or, how about animation? Can you combine animated sequences with real-time, real-people segments for a polished professional look?

Yes, you can with a *digital nonlinear system*. On your own PC, you can be a video god. For the cost of one eight-hour day in a postproduction studio ($3,500 to $4,000), you can buy a multimedia computer capable of handling highly sophisticated video software that allows you to do everything the pros do. For example, on a Packard Bell 166 MHz (Megahertz or "speed of operation"), 16 MB RAM (megabytes, random access memory or "operating memory"), and a 2.5 gigabyte hard drive (actual storage space), you can run several inexpensive commercial digital software programs combining sound, real-time video, and graphics.

Digital video and editor programs allow you to cut and paste video clips, load new video from your camcorder, and dub music in real time to accompany video segments. Digitized frames move around freely like graphic programs such as *Pagemaker*. Once your original masterpiece is ready, you can unload your digital document

(AVI file) onto a VCR tape, and play it back to look like a TV-quality movie.

But don't hold your breath for an Emmy Award. Revolutionary changes in digital editor software are impressive but not equal to what you see on television. There are several reasons for this. First, digital videos are small and require larger hardware boards that produce full-screen movies. Hardware costs for this top-line quality are thousands upon thousands of dollars and not even constructed for PC users. Second, the video medium is cumbersome. When you edit in different video clips, some clips may "miss a beat" in the transfer from videocamera to digital software, and frames may be lost or dropped. In a sequence of 100 frames, if ten frames are dropped during a cut and paste, the remaining 90 frames result in a playback that looks uneven and slightly disjointed. More expensive memory expanders and tinkering with your software program may lower frame-dropping rates. Still, don't expect perfection.

One thing is certain, however. *You do bring video and sound alive on your computer.* Despite current setbacks, digital and editor software programs such as *Microsoft Video for Windows* or *Video Artist* are incredibly cost-efficient and represent the future do-it-yourself technology for homegrown moviemakers. Outputs largely resemble tapes edited in postproduction studios and crafted by industry experts. Now you can copy the experts using the right hardware, affordable software, and just the right mixture of imagination and reality.

AUTHOR'S CORNER

Below is a summary of questionnaire replies from commercial and educational scriptwriters who kindly shared their insights, frustrations, inside gossip, and tips for beginning scribers.

Summary of Replies from Sample Scriptwriters in Mental Health and Allied Fields

1. **Background and degrees:** BAs in videography, filmmaking, psychology, business, education, English, journalism, broad-

casting, editing; MAs in psychology, social work, journalism, filmmaking; PhDs in clinical psychology (few PhDs)

2. **Number of scripts (TV, movie, educational, industrial) sold:** 2 to 10

3. **Number of scripts written but not sold:** 2 to 10; most written on assignment by industrial or infomercial company. Scripts written on spec usually did not sell but provided a sample of author's scriptwriting style.

4. **Average number of pages in scripts submitted:** 30 to 120 pages. Thirty pages for short training and infomercial spots; 120 pages for feature length.

5. **Lag time between submission and acceptance:** two days to two months. Respondents unanimously agreed that interested producers reply in days, not months. A month lag time is a good predictor of disinterest.

6. **Lag time between acceptance and production:** one to two years

7. **Range of advance you receive upon acceptance:** $100 to $5,000 for scripts bought on option, against larger amounts ($3,000 to $10,000) or points (3 percent to 5 percent).

8. **Tips offered to newcomers in scriptwriting:**

   a. It's a very long process. Take your time and write more than one script.
   b. Absolutely persevere.
   c. Producers always need material. Writers on the payroll are becoming too expensive, and hiring trends are favorable for freelancers.

RESOURCES

What makes you a best-selling scriptwriter? Creative story line development? Johnny-on-the-spot rewriting under pressures of a shooting schedule? Possibly it's your ability to predict consumers' buying splurges and proposals for a sure-winner infomercial. Wherever genius comes from, talented writing is only worth dollars once you effectively market yourself. Career boosts in Hollywood-like circles or even among corporate video producers take time, effort, and careful selection of the ideal publicity machine. Brand-name status is not an overnight sensation.

Even if you remain unknown, prolific paying jobs can earn you a part-time or full-time salary working directly out of your house anywhere in the United States. That's the beauty of scriptwriting: it's a home-based job. How serious your efforts reach beyond your house is entirely up to you. One way is slowly to test the freezing waters. Or, you may progress at warp speed once you undertake one or two projects and find them thoroughly enjoyable.

As we've seen, exposure of your gifted scriptwriting abilities lies in self-marketing (Ames, 1996; Aronson and Spetner, 1995). Media relations build recognition by how fast and furious you pitch your ideas to the right sources. Paying a publicist to do this for you is one way. But, as I said earlier, why bother? Costs are so astronomical and career delays so hideous, why sink your savings into a lost cause? Be your own public relations firm.

Advertise strengths in your scripting and promote product ideas with irresistible hooks. Either by fax or e-mail, build a press release kit including biographical sketch, writing credits, and ideas that hype you just enough without overkill. Your press release may in truth have only ten seconds to impress producers before either he or she responds or jump-shoots it into the garbage. So, 99 percent of the time, press releases and pitches kept brief and right on target with consumer needs will get positive replies. The other 1 percent is left for unprepared scripters, betting a longshot on win, place, and show.

To get started, begin with the three resource lists in Chapter 9. The first is a series of training and industrial video producers. Contact these people if your interest lies in writing educational and corporate movies. Following that is a list of infomercial and commercial video producers. Fax these producers with product pitches and queries for freelance infomercial writers. Third, once you have a TV proposal, demo tape from a pilot episode, or financial commitment from investors for taping a pilot show, contact the list of current and to-be-aired cable channels.

Fourth, connect on-line to any number of fantastic websites by the Hollywood Creative Directory (http://hollyvision.com). This is your secret doorway to talent sources. Enjoy weekly updates on key resources in the entertainment field. For a small charge, you can review and download databases on agents and managers, movie studios, networks and producers, film and TV distributors, business and legal personnel, and film and TV music executives.

REFERENCES

Ames, C. (1996). Flirting with P.R.: Telling the Writer's Story. *The Journal of the Writer's Guild of America, 9,* 14-20.

Aronson, M. and Spetner, D. (1995). *The public relations writer's handbook.* Los Angeles, CA: Jossey-Bass.

Hampe, B. (1993). *Video scriptwriting: How to write for the four billion dollar commercial video market.* New York: NAL/Dutton.

Honthaner, E.L. (1993). *The complete film production handbook.* Los Angeles, CA: Lone Eagle Publishing Company.

Kulakow, A. (1996). You don't have to be Jewish, but if you're a young screenwriter, it doesn't hurt. *Moment: Magazine of Jewish Culture and Opinion, 21,* 43.

Litwak, M. (1994). *Contracts for the film and television industry.* Los Angeles, CA: Silman-James Press.

Morley, J. (1992). *Scriptwriting for the impact videos: Imaginative approaches to delivering factual information.* New York: Wadsworth Press.

Ruben, D.H. (1996). *Publicity for mental health clinicians: Using TV, radio, and print media to enhance your public image.* Binghamton, NY: The Haworth Press, Inc.

Wiese, M. (1992). *Film and video financing.* Studio City, CA: Michael Wiese Productions.

Chapter 9

Resources

As mentioned in Chapters 4, 5, 6, 7, and 8, this chapter includes resources for you to use as you seek new ways to make money. This chapter includes information on book publishers, popular magazines, software companies, and television producers.

BOOK PUBLISHERS

Each entry follows a sequence of information based on the replies from each publisher. Entirely completed entries include these items:

Name of Publisher: address, city, state, zip code; fax number; phone number; e-mail or URL (web page) address; Editor/publisher; date established; number of manuscripts submitted per year (mss/yr.); number of titles published per year (titles/yr.); advances/royalty/retail or wholesale; Types of nonfiction books published; Tips for authors and properties needed.

Abbott, Langer & Associates: 48 First Street, Crete, IL 60417-2199; 708-672-4200; Dr. Steven Langer, Publisher; est: 1967; 25 mss/yr; 25 titles/yr; 10-15%/retail; How-to and technical on different phases of human resource management, with few titles specialized for marketing and security management owners.

Accent on Living: PO Box 700, Bloomington, IL 61702; 309-378-4420; 309-378-2961; Betty Garee, Editor; 150 mss/yr; 4 titles/yr.; 6%/retail or outright; Anything dealing with the adjustment process of physically disabled.

ACS Publications: 5521 Ruffin Road, San Diego, CA 92123; 619-492-9919; Maritha Pottenger, Editorial Director; 200 mss/yr; 20 titles/yr; 10-15%/wholesale; Focus on astrology and self-help with themes of self-empowerment.

Active Parenting Publishers Inc.: 810 B Franklin Court, Marietta, GA 30067; 770-429-0334 (fax); CService@activeparenting.com;http://www.activeparenting.com;

Shelly Cox, Editorial Manager; 25 mss/yr; 4 titles/yr; 6-10%/retail; Self-help and esteem-building for parent education, child rearing, psychology, and family issues.

Adams Media Corporation: 260 Center Street, Holbrook, MA 02343; 617-767-0994; 617-767-8100; http://www.adamsonline.com; Edward Waltels, Editor in Chief; est: 1980; 1,000 mss/yr; 50 titles/yr; variable; Self-esteem, psychology, business and careers, with focus on impulse purchasers.

Adams-Blake Publishing: 8041 Sierra Street; Fair Oaks, CA 95628; 916-962-9296; Monica Blane, Senior Editor; 90 mss/yr; 10-15 titles/yr; 10%/whole-sale; How-to and technical that is easily sold to businesses and industry on money, medicine, health, economics, electronics, or directly related to workforce.

Addicus Books, Inc: PO Box 37327; Omaha, NE 68137; Rod Colvin, President; 4 to 5 titles/yr; Self-help on true crime, economics, medicine and health, and business. Focus on research-based materials.

Allen Publishing Company: 7324 Reseda Blvd., Reseda CA; 91335; 818-344-6788; Michael Wiener, Publisher; est: 1979; 100 mss/yr; 4 titles/yr; outright; Focused on wealth and opportunity seekers, aspiring entrepreneurs, specializing in materials for people with little capital for business start-up but who are motivated.

Alpine Publications Inc: 225 S. Madison Avenue, Loveland, CO; 80537-6514; 303-667-9317; B.J. McKinney, Publisher; est: 1975; 6 titles/yr; 7-15%/retail; Devotes press to dog breeding and training books for AKC readers, focusing on guidebooks for animal lovers.

Alyson Publications: 40 Plympton Street, Boston, MA 02118-2425; 213-467-6805; 213-871-1225; Tom Radko, Publisher; est: 1979; 500 mss/yr; 30 titles/yr; 8-15%/retail; Looking for new authors on raising kids by lesbian and gay parents plus nonfiction on gay/lesbian subjects on self-help for nonacademic readers.

Amacom Books: American Management Association, 135 W. 50th Street, New York, NY 10020-1201; 212-903-8081; Weldon P. Rackley, Managing Director; est: 1923; 200 mss/yr; 68 titles/yr; 10-15%/retail; Publishing arm of American Management Association covering practical books on college, corporate markets, technology, professional skills.

America West Publishers: PO Box 3300, Bozeman, MT 59772-3300; 406-585-0703; 406-585-0700; George Green, Review Editor; est: 1985; 150 mss/yr; 20 titles/yr; $300 advance; 10%/retail; Mainstream nonfiction on UFOs, metaphysical, holistic, political cover-up, and controversy.

Andrews and McMeel: 4900 Main Street, Kansas City, MO 64112; 816-932-6700; Christine Schillig, Vice President; est: 1933; Offers general trade nonfiction and consumer reference with focus on children's issues and books for kids.

Arcade Publishing: 141 Fifth Avenue, New York, NY 10010; 212-475-2633; Richard Seaver, Publisher; est: 1988; 40 titles/yr; $1,000-$10,000 advance; Looking for general topics on cooking, foods, history, government, politics, self-help.

Avery Publishing Group: 120 Old Broadway, Garden City Park, NY 11040; 516-742-1892; 516-741-2155; Managing editor; est: 1976; 200-300 mss/yr; 40 titles/yr; 10%/wholesale; How-to in business, economics, childrearing, health and medicine, military and war

Avon Books: 1350 Avenue of the Americas, New York, NY 10019; Alice Webster-Williams; est: 1941; 400 titles/yr; negotiable; Popular psychology, self-help, history, health, economics, and politics.

Baker Book House Company: PO Box 6287; Grand Rapids, MI 49516-6287; 616-676-9573; 616-675 9185; postmaster@bakerbooks.com; see web page at http://www.bakerbooks.com; Jane Schrier, Acquisitions; est: 1939; 1,500-2,000 mss/yr; 200 titles/yr; 14%/retail; Self-help, parenting guidance, ministry tools, and trade books that combine personal testimony with current issues through Christian perspective.

Ballantine Books: 201 E. 50th Street, New York, NY 10022; 212-572-2149; Pamela Strickler, Senior Editor; Cadillac firm specializing in mass market and trade paperback on parenting, health and medicine, self-improvement.

Bantam Books: Dept. WM, 1540 Broadway, New York, NY 10036; 212-782-9523; 212-354-6500; Ms. Toni Burbank, Editor; est: 1945; 350 titles/yr; negotiable; Top firm producing biography, how-to, humor, self-help, parenting, diet, psychology, gay/lesbian, and general mainstream areas for commercial market.

Bell Tower: Crown Publishing, 201 E. 50th Street, New York, NY 10022; 212-572-2051; Toinette Lippe, Editorial Director; 9 titles/yr; negotiable; Spiritual self-help, gift books, health and wellness, with sharp marketing focus on bible gift stores.

Berkley Publishing Group: 200 Madison Avenue. New York, NY 10016; 212-545-8917; 212-951-8800; Leslie Gelbman, Editor-in-Chief; 800 titles/yr; How-to books pertaining to family, life, business, health, nutrition, crime, military.

Berrett-Koehler Publishers: 155 Montgomery Street, San Francisco, CA 94104-4109; 415-288-0260; Steve Piersanti, President; est: 1992; Books on career development, entrepreneurship, human resources, management, leadership, office politics.

Blue Dolphin Publishing Inc.: PO Box 1920, Nevada City, CA 95959-1920; 916-265-0787; 916-265-6925; bdolphin@netshel.net; Christopher Comins, Mass Market Editor; est: 1985; 3,000 mss/yr; 12-15 titles/yr; 10-15%/wholesale; Specializes in books in comparative spirituality and transpersonal psychology, self-help, healing, and self-growth with conscious evolution theme.

Blue Star Productions: Bookworld, 9666 E Riggs Road, #194 Sun Lakes, AZ 85248; 602-895-7995; Barbara DeBolt, Editor; 500 mss/yr; 10-12 titles/yr;

10%/wholesale; Mass market on philsophy, ufology, metaphysical, new age, and time travel, with Native American themes also accepted.

Bonus Books, Inc.: 160 E. Illinois Street, Chicago, IL 60611; 312-467-0580; http.//www.bonusbooks.com; Deborah Flapan, Managing Editor; est: 1985; 400-500 mss/yr; 30 titles/yr; 10%/retail; Biography, how-to on business, economics, foods, nutrition, health, medicine, recreation, true crime.

Brighton Publications Inc: PO Box 120706, St. Paul, MN 55112-0706; 612-636-2220; Sharon E. Dlugosch, Editor; 20 mss/yr; 4 titles/yr; 10%/wholesale; How-to business and coffee-table and party themes on any topic relevant to dialogue interest in groups.

Business McGraw-Hill: 11 W. 19th Street,New York, NY 10011; 212-337-5999; 212-337-4098; Philip Ruppel, Publisher; est: 1969; 1,200 mss/yr; 100 titles/yr; $1,000-$100,000 advance; 5-17%/retail; How-to reference and self-help in business marketplace emphasizing money, finance, government, politics, and capability of writer to be promoter.

Cambridge Educational: PO Box 2153, Charleston, WV 25328-2153; 304-744-9351; 800-468-4227; Edward T. Gardner, PhD, President; est: 1980; 200 mss/yr; 12 titles/yr; $1,500-$4,000 outright; Educational publisher for young (13-24 years old) readers on job search, career guidance, money, finance, parenting, food nutrition, physical education, health, with books sold to schools and libraries.

Camino Books, Inc.: PO Box 59026, Philadelphia, PA 19102; 215-732-2491; E. Jutkowitz, Publisher; est: 1987; 500 mss/yr; 5 titles/yr; $1,000 advance; 6-12%/retail; Focus for Middle Atlantic States covering child guidance and parenting, cooking, foods, ethnic, gardening, Americana, government, history, and regional activities.

Capra Press: PO Box 2068, Santa Barbara, CA 93210; 805-966-4590; Noel Young, President; est: 1970; List includes mainstream on nature, natural history, mystery, travel, postcard series.

Cardoza Publishing: 132 Hastings Street, Brooklyn, NY 11235; 718-743-5229; Rose Swann, Acquisitions Editor; 70 mss/yr; 175 titles/yr; $500-$2,000 advance; 15-20%/retail; Imprints reflect entire focus on gaming, gambling, health and fitness, world travel, and competition. Also looking for multimedia expansions.

Career Assurance Press: PO Box 12695, Scottsdale, AZ 85267-2695; 602-998-2173; 602-998-9411; capress1@aol.com; Larry James, Editor; est: 1992; 2 mss/yr; 2 titles/yr; Catalog boasts business, personal relationships, and upbeat contemporary topics for romance-possible subsidy.

Career Press: PO Box 687, Franklin Lakes, NJ 07417; 201-848-0310; Ronald Fry, President; est: 1985; Highlights career path on practical business books, financial planning, how-to resume, retirement, and job searching strategies.

Carol Publishing: 120 Enterprise Ave., Secaucus, NJ, 07094; 201-866-8159; 201-866-0490; Steve Schragis, Publisher; est: 1985; 2,000 mss/yr; 180 titles/yr;

$1,000 advance; 5-15%/retail; General commercial mass trade on humor, self-help, business, computers, cooking, military and war, women's issues.

Carroll & Graf Publishers: 260 Fifth Avenue, New York, NY 10001; 212-889-8772; Kent Carroll, Publisher; est: 1983; Produces topics on business, true crime, contemporary culture, current events, self-improvement for mainstream groups.

Cassandra Press: PO Box 868, San Rafael, CA 94915; 415-382-7758; 415-382-8507; Gurudas, President; est: 1986; 200 mss/yr; 6 titles/yr; 6-8%/retail; New age, how-to, self-help, metaphysical themes in holistic fields.

Christian Publications, Inc.: 3825 Hartzdalle Drive, Camp Hill, PA 17011; 717-761-7044; David E. Fesenden, Editor; 400 mss/yr; varies; Christian and missionary denomination covering family and marriage, self-help with deeper personal growth themes.

Chronimed Publishing: 13911 Ridgedale Drive, Suite 250, Minneapolis, MN 55343; 612-541-0239; David Wexler, Associate Producer; Features life-enhancing breathroughs on self-improvement, fitness and health, eating, coping with chronic illness, and books on diabetes.

Citadel Press: 120 Enterprise, Secaucus, NJ 07094; 201-866-8159 (fax); Allan J. Wilson, Editorial Director; est: 1945; 800-1,000 mss/yr; 60-80 titles/yr; $5,000 advance; 5-7%/retail; Concentrates on popular genres from film and self-help to humor, history, and off-beat material.

Cliff/Fay Institute Inc.: 2207 Jackson Street, Golden, CO 80401; 303-278-7552; Nancy M. Henry, President; 18 titles/yr; $500-$5,000 advance; 5-7%/retail; Self-help topics on parental guidance, education, health and medicine, sociology, psychology, social trends. No personal stories or new age.

Conari Press: 2550 North St., Suite 101, Berkeley, CA 94710; 510-649-7175; Mary Jane Ryan, Executive Editor; est: 1987; 800 mss/yr; 17 titles/yr; $1,500 advance; 8-12%/retail; Psychology and self-help categories with bent toward spirituality, women's issues. Looking for proposals with targeted audience.

Consortium Publishing: 640 Weaver Hill Road, West Greenwich, RI 02817-2261; John Carlevale, Publisher; est: 1990; 25 mss/yr; 10-12 titles/yr; Trade paperback line in psychology, self-help, childcare, science, education, health and medicine, with limited first print runs.

Consumer Reports Books: 101 Truman Avenue, Yonkers, NY 10703-1057; 914-378-2904 (fax); Mark Hoffman; est: 1936; 500 mss/yr; 15-20 titles/yr; How-to and reference on product update, assessment, including medicine, health, home owner's needs, money and finance. Tailored for budget and safety-minded consumer.

Contemporary Books, Inc.: Two Prudential Plaza, Suite 1200, Chicago, IL 60601; 312-540-4657; 312-540-4500; Nancy J. Crossman, Editorial Director; est: 1947; 2,500 mss/yr; 75 titles/yr; 6-15%/retail; Mainstream nonfiction trade on self-help, business, finance, health and fitness, psychology, sports, real estate, nutrition, popular culture, women's studies.

Crisp Publications, Inc.: 1200 Hamilton Ct, Menlo Park, CA 94025-1427; 415-323-6100; Michael G. Crisp, Publisher; est: 1985; 25-30 titles/yr; Focus on business, economics, money, and finance, with self-help line in medicine and health.

Crossing Press: 97 Hanger Way, Watsonville, CA 95019; Elaine Goldman; est: 1972; 1,600 mss/yr; 50 titles/yr; Subjects recently include cookbooks, simple how-to's on health and self-esteem, women's interests, new age, gender and gay issues.

Cypress Publishing Group: 11835 ROE #187, Leawood, KS 66211; 913-681-9875; Carl Heintz, VP, Marketing; 10 titles/yr; 10-15%/wholesale; Currently looking for self-help in technical, hobbies, electronics, software, illustrated books, business, economics, pushing high-profile book sales.

Dancing Jester Press: 3411 Garth Road, Suite 208, Baytown, TX 77521; 713-428-8685; 713-427-9560; djpress@aol.com; Glenda Daniel, Editor; 20 titles/yr; 4-12%/retail or outright; Autobiography, children/juvenile, coffeee table book, how-to with focus on nutrition, ethnic, lesbian, health and medicine, and psychology. Recent push is toward software adaptations.

Dartnell Corporation: 4660 North Ravenswood Avenue, Chicago, IL 60640; 312-561-4000; Scott B. Pemberton, VP, editorial division; est: 1917; Business information publisher known for motivational customer service, teamwork, and gender-based office-strategy line.

Delphi Press, Inc.: PO Box 267990, Chicago, IL 60626; 312-274-7912; 312-274-7910; Karen Jackson, Publisher; est: 1989; 20-30 mss/yr; 10-12 titles/yr; 7-12%/wholesale; Focus on women's spirituality, men's supernaturalism including wicca, witchcraft, pagan practice, ritual healing, divination, nature and earth religions, deep ecology, and sacred psychology.

Dimi Press: 3820 Oak Hollow Lane, SE Salem,OR; 97302-4774; 503-364-9727; 503-364-7698; dickbook@aol.com; Dick Lutz, Editor; est: 1981; 50-75 mss/yr; 4-5 titles/yr; 10%/retail; How-to books on childcare, adolescents, parenting, living in comporary society, with focus on practical and school-based issues.

Discus Press: 3389 Sheridan Street, #308, Hollywood, FL 33021; 305-963-7134; Karen Weiss, Senior Editor; 5 titles/yr; $2,500-$10,000 advance; 10-12%/retail; Searching for biography, health and medicine, psychology, history, education, agriculture, women's issues, and variety of other topics along self-help lines.

Distinctive Publishing Corporation: PO Box 17868, Plantation, FL 33318-7868; 305-975-2413; 305-975-2413; C. Pierson, Editor; est: 1986; 1,200 mss/yr; 25 titles/yr; 6-10%/retail; Wide-range coverage of trade how-to's on health and medicine, psychology, sociology, education, parenting.

Donald I. Fine, Inc.: 19 W. 21st Street, New York, NY 10010; 212-366-2933; 212-366-2570; Donald Fine, Publisher; est: 1983; 1,000 mss/yr; 45-60 titles/yr;

Generic; Publisher shifting from self-help to more history, sports, military, and contemporary issues.

Doral Publishing Inc.: 8560 SW Salish Lane #300, Wilsonville, OR 97070-9625; 503-682-2648; 503-682-3307; Luana Luther, Editor-in-Chief; 12 mss/yr; 7 titles/yr; 10-17%/wholesale; Outlet publisher on purebred dogs covering how-to, reference, for kids and adult pet owners, trainers.

Doubleday: 1540 Broadway, New York, NY 10036; 212-354-6500; Elizabeth Lerner, Editor; est: 1897; Rolls Royce publisher drawing revered authors and paying higher advances based on author track record, pre-saleability of book, and topics on current events, psychology, health, medicine, education, politics, celebrities.

Drama Books Publisher: 260 Fifth Avenue, New York, NY 10001; 212-725-8506; 212-725-5377; dramapub@interport.net; http://www.interport.net ~dramapub; Ina Kohler, Managing Editor; est: 1967; 420 mss/yr; 4-15 titles/yr; negotiable; Premier publisher of performing arts self-help books, directories, reference, manuals highlighting theory, practice for actors, directors, producers, management, in radio, TV, cable, playwriting, criticism, and reviews thereof.

Dutton/Signet: 375 Hudson Street, New York, NY 10014; 212-366-2000; Elaine Koster, Publisher; est: 1852; 90 titles/yr; Popular press leader in self-help, serious nonfiction, and psychology books.

Ecco Press: 100 W. Broad Street, Hopewell, NJ 08525; 609-466-4748; Daniel Halpern, Editor-in-Chief; est: 1970; 40 titles/yr; $250-$1,000 advance; 7-12%/retail; Rising company in coffee table books on government, politics, food and nutrition, language, literature, military, cooking.

Elder Books: PO Box 490 , Forest Knolls, CA 94933; 415-488-9002; Carmel Sheridan, Director; 50 mss/yr; 6-10 titles/yr; $500-2,000 advance; 7%/retail; Original trades on health, medicine, religion, psychology, all toward senior issues.

Elysium Growth Press: 5436 Fernwood Avenue, Los Angeles, CA 90027; 310-455-2007; 310-455-1000; 20 mss/yr; 4 titles/yr; $3,000 advance; retail Niche publisher focused on nudity, naturalism, body self-image and self-appreciation depicting the clothing-optional lifestyle.

Enslow Publishers Inc.: 44 Fadem Road, PO Box 699, Springfield, NJ 07081; 201-379-8890; Brian D. Enslow, Publisher; est: 1977; 90 titles/yr; Strongly seeking nonfiction for young adults and children in areas of social, biography, recreation, and science.

EPM Publications Inc.: BOX 490, McLean, VA 22101; Evelyn P. Metzger, Publisher; 8-10 titles/yr; 6-15%/retail; Smaller publisher focusing on biography, child guidance, how-to, self-help, military (civil war), women's issues.

M. Evans and Co., Inc.: 216 E. 49th Street, New York, NY 10017; 212-486-4544; 212-688-2810; Bette Ann Crawford, Editor; est: 1960; 30-40 titles/yr;

negotiable; General trade focusing on quality commercial potential in health and behavioral sciences but open to other subjects.

Faber & Faber, Inc.: 50 Cross Street,Winchester, MA 01890; 617-729-2783; 617-721-1427; Adrian Wood, Editorial Assistant; est: 1976; 1,200 mss/yr; 30 titles/yr; Trend toward popular culture, serious intelligent rock-and-roll books/ anthologies with bent on field, screenplays, history, and natural history.

Firebrand Books: 141 The Commons, Ithaca, NY; 14850; 607-272-0000; Nancy Bereano, Publisher; est:1985; 400-500 mss/yr; 8-10 titles/yr; 7-9%/retail; Personal narratives reflecting feminism and lesbian lifestyle.

Fisher Books: 4239 W. Ina Road, Suite 101, Tucson, AZ 85741; 602-744-0944; 602-744-6110; Editorial Submissions Director; est: 1987; 16 titles/yr; 10-15%/wholesale; Subjects include automotive, cooking and food, gardening, family health, self-esteem.

J. Flores Publications: PO Box 830131, Miami, FL 33283-0131; Eli Flores, Editor; est: 1982; 10 titles/yr; Special interest on careers, business, and consumer-consciousness.

Floricanto Press: 16161 Ventura Blvd, Suite 830, Encino, CA 91436; 818-990-1879; 6 titles/yr; 5%/wholesale; Specialty publisher for Hispanic readers on health, medicine, history, anthropology, psychology, popular self-help topics.

Free Spirit Publishing: 400 First Avenue North, Suite 616, Minneapolis, MN 55401; 612-338-2068; Elizabeth Verdick, Editor; est: 1983; 15-20 titles/yr; 5-12%/retail; Features education guides for students, educators, parents, and mental health organizations, including self-help for these populations with special education as focus.

Fulcrum Publishing: 350 Indiana Street, Suite 350, Golden, CO 80401; 303-277-1623; T.J.Baker, Acquisitions Editor; est: 1984; Book selections diversifying to nature and outdoors, business, travel guides, and educational books for children and adults.

Gardner Press, Inc.: 6801 Lake Worth Road, #104, Lake Worth, FL 33467; 407-964-9700; 407-964-9700; G. Spungin, Publisher; 200 mss/yr; 20 titles; 5-10%/wholesale; Promotes biography, self-help in psychology, sociology, women's issues, nature, and books showing high presales potential.

Garrett Publishing: 384 South Military Trail, Deerfield Beach, FL 33442; 305-480-8543; Debra L. Franco, Editorial Manager; est: 1990; 15 mss/yr; 10 titles/yr; 10-15%/wholesasle; Focuses on business, finance, law, and personal budget, but style is with practical, ready-to-use templates, sample forms, checklists, instructions, informative examples for immediate application.

Gay Sunshine Press: PO Box 410690, San Francisco, CA 94141-0690; Winston Leyland, Editor; est: 1970; 6-8 titles/yr; outright or retail; Exclusive focus on how-to and gay lifestyles dealing with contemporary and psychological perspectives of practical life.

General Publishing: 2701 Ocean Park Blvd., Suite 140, Santa Monica, CA 90405; 310-314-4000; Peter Hoffman, Managing Editor; est: 1991; Emphasizes celebrity and media-oriented general interest works used as gift books or autobiography editions for mass market.

Glenbridge Publishing, Ltd.: 6010 W. Jewell Avenue, Denver, CO 80232-7106; 303-987-9037 (fax); James A. Keene, Editor; est: 1986; 6-8 titles/yr; 10%/retail; General subjects of trade nonfiction covered, with interest in business, economics, psychology, and social history.

Gylantic Publishing Company: PO Box 2792, Littleton, CO 80161-2792; 303-727-4279; 303-797-6093; Julie Baker, Editor; est: 1991; 600 mss/yr; 5 titles/yr; 7-12%/retail; Innovative interests in parenting, young adult (men/women's) issues with social impact.

Hampton Roads Publishing Company Inc.: 976 Norfolk Square, Norfolk, VA 23502-3209; 804-455-8907; 804-459-2453; Robert S. Friedman, Publisher; est: 1989; 325 mss/yr; 20 titles/yr; 8-15%/wholesale; Rising publisher in self-help metaphysics and new age disciplines for mainstream readership.

Harcourt Brace & Company: 525 B Street, Suite 1900, San Diego, CA; 619-231-6616; Vick Austin-Smith, Senior Editor-San Diego; est: 1919; Giant industry leader of mainstream nonfiction particularly potent in commercial self-help, education, and special interest. Credentials a must.

Harlan Davidson, Inc: 773 Glenn Avenue, Wheeling, IL 60090-6000; 708-541-9830; 708-541-9720; Maureen G. Hewitt, Editor-in-Chief; est: 1972; 25 mss/yr; 15 titles/yr; Variety of mainstream titles from philsophy and business to history and self-help emphasizing author credentials.

HarperCollins Publishers: 10 East 53rd Street, New York, NY 10022; 212-207-7000; Robert Jones, Senior Editor; est: 1817; Sacrosanct reputation as commanding leader in trade divisions ranging from psychology self-help to business, true crime, finance, and just about any topic.

Hartley & Marks: PO Box 147, Point Roberts, WA 98281; 206-945-2017; Vic Marks, Editorial Director; est: 1973; 8-10 titles/yr; 7-10%/retail; How-to, self-help on building healthy lifestyles through practical solutions using psychology, holistic medicine, nature, and environment.

Harvard Common Press: 535 Albany Street, Boston, MA 02118-2500; 617-423-0679; 617-423-5803; Dan Rosenberg, Managing Editor; est: 1976; 1,000 mss/yr; 8 titles/yr; Line nearly entirely is parenting and childcare books, helping people gain control over their lives.

Harvest House Publishers: 1075 Arrowsmith, Eugene, OR 97402-9197; 503-342-6410; 503-343-0123; LaRae Weikert, Manager; est: 1974; 3,500 mss/yr; 70-80 titles/yr; 14-18%/wholesale; Self-help covering women's and family issues within evangelical Christian orientation.

Hastings House: 141 Halstead Avenue, Mamaroneck, NY 10543-2652; 914-835-1037; 914-835-40095; Hy Steirman, Editor; 125 mss/yr; 12 titles/yr; 8-10%/retail;

Shifting focus to coffee table and self-help in health and medicine, psychology, travel, and consumer needs.

Hatherleigh Press: 420 E. 51st St., New York, NY 10022; 212-308-7930; 212-355-0882; Frederic Flach, Editor-in-Chief; est: 1992; 20 mss/yr; 12 titles/yr, 10-15%/retail/outright; Recovery and self-help books for mental health market from AIDS to technical counseling manuals.

Hawkes Publishing Inc.: 5947 South 350 West, Murray, UT 84107; 801-266-5599; 801-266-5555; Shanna J. Smith, Editor; est: 1965; 200 mss/yr; 24 titles/yr; 10%/wholesale; Catalog shows cooking, foods, health, and history, how-to and self-help topics based on how marketably promising the manuscript is.

Haworth Press: 10 Alice Street, Binghamton, NY 13904-1580; 607-722-5857; Bill Palmer, Managing Editor; est: 1973; 150 mss/yr; 60 titles/yr; 8-10%/retail; Reference and trade publisher lately expanding line to wider consumer market with imprints covering psychology, health/medicine, gay/lesbian, religion, nursing, pharmacy, food services, women's studies, international business.

Hay House, Inc.: PO Box 6204, Carson, CA 90749-6204; 310-605-0601; Jill Kramer, Editorial Director; est: 1985; 900 mss/yr; 12 titles/yr; up to $5,000 advance; 8-10%/retail; Primarly self-help on ecology, nutrition, education, health, medicine, psychology and new age, all having positive slant for personal improvement.

Health Communications, Inc.: 3201 Southwest 15th Street, Deerfield Beach, FL 33442; 305-360-0909 (fax); 102450.722@compjserve.com; http.//www.pur.com/hci/; Christine Belleris, Acquisitions Editor; est: 1976; 30 titles/yr; 15-20%/retail; Growing popularity as hottest selling book line on recovery, addictions, personal regrowth, and spiritual formation.

Health Press: PO Box 1388, Santa Fe, NM 87504; 505-983-1733; 505-982-9373; K. Schwartz, Publisher; 80 mss/yr; 4 titles/yr wholesale; Patient education manuals and books on health, medicine, self-help authored by professionals.

Henry Holt & Company: 115 West 18th Street, New York, NY 10011; 212-886-9200; Cynthia Vartan, Editor at large; est: 1866; Draws exceptional authors on family-oriented and popular self-help books and consumer guides.

Honor Books, Inc.: PO Box 5388, Tulsa, OK 74155; 918-496-9007; Krista Dalrymple, Acquisitions; 30 titles/yr; 5-15%/wholesale; Christian perspective offered on parenting, family issues, guidebooks on biblical wisdom, money and finance.

Houghton Mifflin Company: 222 Berkely Street, Boston, MA 02116-3764; 617-725-5000; Richard Todd, Editor; est: 1832; Grand tradition of marketing imprints on travel, self-improvement, travel, religion, biography, and science.

Human Services Institute, Inc.: 165 W. 91st Street, Suite 7-H, New York, NY 10024-1357; 212-769-9738; Dr. Lee Marvin Joiner, Senior Editor; est: 1988; 100

mss/yr; 10-12 titles/yr; 7-15%/wholesale; Sells to hospitals, clinics, mental health centers, and looking for childcare, parenting, self-help on variety of topics.

Hunter House Publishers: PO Box, 2914, Alameda, CA 94501-0914; 510-865-4295; 510-865-5282; ordering@hunterhouse.com; Ms. Lisa E. Lee, editor; 100 mss/yr.; 12 titles/yr; 0-$3,000 advance; 12%/retail; Emerging publisher in trade market targets savvy, educated readers, mostly women, seeking real-life issues on sexuality, violence prevention, teaching, wellness, health, gay and lesbian, and relationships. Recently expanded line in self-help.

ICS Books, Inc: 1370 E. 86th Place, Merrillville, IN 46410; 216-769-0585; Thomas A. Todd, Editor; 8-10 titles/yr; 10%/wholesale; Trade paperbacks include health, nature, recreation, how-to self-improvement and women's issues.

Ide House Publishers: 4631 Harvey Drive, Mesquite, TX 75150; 214-686-5332; Ryan Idol, President; 500 mss/yr; 10 titles/yr; 7%/retail; Women's history, gay/lesbian but writing must be nonsexist, nonhomophobic; Transition from being scholarly house.

ILR Press: Cornell University Press, Sage House, 512 E. State Street, Ithaca, NY 14850; 607-277-2374; 607-277-2338; E. Benson, Editor; est: 1945; 12-15 titles/yr; Expressly interested in manuscripts in industrial and labor relations for general public.

Inner Traditions International: PO Box 388, 1 Park Street, Rochester, VT 05767; 802-767-3726; 802-767-3174; Ms. Lee Wood, Acquisitions Editor; est: 1975; 2,000 mss/yr; 40 titles/yr; $1,000 advance; 8-10%/retail; Spiritual, new age approach on alternative medicine, mythology, indigenous cultures, esoteric philosophy, psychology, transpersonal theory, showing personal transformation.

International Wealth Success: PO Box 186, Merrick, NY 11570-0186; 516-766-5919; 516-766-5850; Tyler G. Hicks, Editor; est: 1967; 100 mss/yr; 10 titles/yr; 10%/wholesale; Self-help techniques inspire building wealth, financing, business, success, venture capital, and developing entrepreneurship.

Jist Works, Inc: 720 N. Park Avenue, Indianapolis, IN 46202-3431; 317-264-3709; 317-264-3720; jistworks@aol.com; Sara Hall, Managing Editor; est: 1981; 300 mss/yr; 5-12%/wholesale; Push is for trades in how-to, career, helping to guide professional and educated readers.

LangMarc Publishing: PO Box 33817, San Antonio, TX 78265-3817; 210-822-5014; 210-822-2521; Langmarc@aol.com; Dr. James Qualben, Editor; est: 1990; 3-5 titles/yr; Thriving publisher of inspirational, religious self-help, and reference topics.

Larson Publications: 4936 Route 414, Burdett, NY 14818-9729; 607-546-9342; Paul Cash, Director; est: 1982; 1,000 mss/yr; 4-5 titles/yr; 7%/retail; Sells spiritual philsophy with new age edge, including self-help psychology, religion, and transsectarian viewpoints.

Libra Publishers, Inc.: 3089C Clairemont Drive, Suite 383, San Diego, CA 92117-6892; 619-571-1414; William Kroll, Publisher; est: 1960; 300 mss/yr; 15

titles/yr; 10-15%/retail; Multi-genre books given consideration but emphasis is on simple how-to's in behavioral sciences.

Lifetime Books, Inc.: 2131 Hollywood Blvd., Hollywood, FL 33020; 305-925-5244; 305-925-5242; Brian Feinblum, Senior Editor; 1,500 mss/yr; 25 titles/yr; $500-$5,000 advance; 6-15%/retail; Strong selling nonfiction trades from business to self-help and parenting to money/finance and biography/expose and true crime. References and professional expertise a plus.

Liguori Publications: One Liguori Drive, Liguori, MO 63057; 314-464-8449; 314-464-2500; Thomas M. Santa, Publisher; 20 titles/yr; 9%/retail; Exploring direction of CD-ROM on self-help devotion, juvenile, and upbeat religious themes.

Little, Brown and Company: 1271 Avenue of the Americas, New York, NY 10020; 212-522-2067; 212-522-8700; Kathrynn Di Tommaso, Editor; est: 1837; 100 titles/yr; A Time-Warner conglomerate publishing a range of mass paperback originals with literary distinction but presales potential for self-help and true crime books.

Llewellyn Publications: PO Box 64383, St. Paul, MN 55164-0383; 612-291-1908; 612-291-1970; Nancy J. Mostad, Acquisitions Manager; est: 1901; 500 mss/yr; 72 titles/yr; 10%/wholesale; Traditional publisher featuring a wide variety of self-help practical guides for health, nutrition, metaphysical, psychology, women's studies, but with a highly entertaining slant.

Loompanics Unlimited: PO Box 1197, Port Townsend, WA 98368-0997; 360-385-7785 (fax); loompanx@well.com; Michael Hoy, President; est: 1975; 500 mss/yr; 15 titles/yr; $500 advance or outright; 10-15%/wholesale; How-to, self-help on drugs, self-sufficiency, espionage, investigation, police methods, and other subjects reflecting matters against the "system."

Love and Logic Press: 2207 Jackson Street, Golden, CO 80401; Nancy Henry, Publisher; 5-12 titles/yr; $500-5,000 advance; 7-12%/wholesale; Small press focusing on child guidance, health, medicine, psychology, and sociology (self-help theme)

Luramedia: PO Box 261668, San Diego, CA 92196-1668; 619-578-7560; 619-578-1948; Lura Jane Geiger, Ph.D., Editorial Director; est: 1982; 500 mss/yr; 6-8-titles/yr; 10%/wholesale; Books on healing, hope, and spiritual promise with underlying biblical theme or personal reflection shown through technique.

MacMurray & Beck: PO Box 150717, Lakewood, CO 80215; Frederick Ramey, Executive Editor; 5-8-titles/yr; $2,000-8,000 outright; 8-12%/retail; Looking for thoughtfully insightful and nonacademic books on health, medicine, men's issues, psychology, personal narratives, women's issues.

Madison Books: 4720 Boston Way, Lanham MD 20706; 301-459-2118; 301-459-3366; Julie Kirsch, Managing Editor; est: 1984; 1,200 mss/yr; 40 titles/yr; 10-15%/retail; Trade publisher covering history, contemporary affairs, psychology, life issues.

Marketscope Books: 119 Richard Court, Aptos, CA 95003; 408-688-7535; Ken Albert, Editor-in-Chief; est: 1985; 10 titles/yr; 10-15%/wholesale; How-to and self-help beat oriented in sexuality, money and finance, psychology, parenting, and hobbies.

Markowski International Publishers: One Oakglade Circle, Hummelstown, PA 17036-9525; 717-566-6423; 717-566-0468; Marjorie L. Markowski, Editor-in-Chief; est: 1981; 500 mss/yr; 12 titles/yr; Primary focus is on popular health, marriage, human relations, personal development with self-help strategy theme increasing sales in business genres.

Mastermedia: 17 E. 89th Street, New York, NY 10128; 212-546-7650; Merry Clark, Director of Marketing; 20 titles/yr; 10-20%/wholesale; Authors are professional speakers whose workshops, training, and media appearances largely boost self-help sales in parenting, psychology, religion, women's issues, and business. Submit evidence showing author is proven expert in field.

Masters Press: 2647 Waterfront Pkwy., Suite 300, Indianapolis, IN 46214-2041; 317-298-5604; 317-298-5706; Holly Kondras, Managing Editor; est: 1986; 50 mss/yr; 30-40 titles/yr; $1,000-5,000 advance; 10-15%/retail; Tailors to sports enthusiasts, people interested in fitness, offering self-help books on recreation, sports, biography.

Merloyd Lawrence Books: Addison-Wesley Publishers, 102 Chestnut Street, Boston, MA 02108; Merloyd Lawrence, President; est: 1982; 400 mss/yr; 8 titles/yr; retail; Majority of subjects center on child development, parenting, health and medicine, psychology.

Mother Courage Press: 1667 Douglas Avenue, Racine WI 53404-2721; 414-637-8242; 414-637-2227; Barbara Lindquist, Publisher; est: 1981; 800-900 mss/yr; 4 titles/yr; $250 advance; 10-15%/wholesale; Popular press highlighting courageous and socially heroic women, with self-help on sexual abuse, psychology, spirituality, Native American women, and lesbianism.

Thomas Nelson Publishers: Nelson Place at Elm Hill Pike, PO Box 141000, Nashville, TN 37214-1000; 615-889-9000; Submissions Editor; est: 1798; 250 titles/yr; Among largest Christian publishers of spiritual self-help and recovery books featuring inspirational and motivational material.

New Falcon Publications: 1739 E. Broadway Road, suite 1-277, Tempe, AZ 85282; 602-708-1409; 602-708-1409; Frank Martin, Editor; est: 1980; 400 mss/yr; 15-20 titles/yr; up to $5,000 advance; 5-15%/retail; Company publishes gay, lesbian, health, medicine, psychology, and archeology subjects with some subsidy (co-venture) if market prospects look slim.

New Harbinger Publications: 5674 Shattuck Avenue, Oakland, CA 94609; 510-652-5472; newharbpub@aol.com;http.//www.newharbinger.com; Kristen Beck, Acquisitions Editor; 200 mss/yr; 16 titles/yr; Looking for qualified psychotherapists writing on practitioner-needed topics in child guidnace, health and medicine, recovery, addiction, and health.

NewMarket Press: 18 East 48th Street, New York, NY 10017; 212-832-3575; Esther Margolis, Publisher; est: 1981; 10 titles/yr; General nonfiction trades in humor, psychology, parenting, nutrition, cooking, personal finance, business, distributed through Random House.

New World Library: 14 Pamaron Way, Novato, CA 94949; 415-884-2199; 415-884-2100; becknwlib.com; Marc Allen, Publisher; 25 titles/yr; $0-$200,000 advance; 12-16%/wholesale; Strong trade paperback house listing self-help, business, money, finance, personal growth, spirituality.

Nova Science Publishers, Inc.: 6080 Jericho Turnpike, Suite 207, Commack, NY 11725-2808; 516-499-3146; 516-499-3103; novascil@aol.com; Frank Columbus, Editor-in-Chief; 1,000 mss/yr; 150 titles/yr; Self-help and textbooks on computers, history, health and medicine, child development, religion, science.

Paper Chase Press: 5721 Magazine Street #152, New Orleans, LA 70115; 504-522-2025; Jennifer Osborn, Editor; 5 titles/yr; retail; How-to and self-help on hobbies, psychology, religion, but authors should be high-profile marketing enthusiasts.

Papier-Mache Press: 135 Aviation Way #14, Watsonville, CA 95076; 408-763-1420; Shirley Coe, Acquisitions Editor; 6-8 titles/yr; $500-$1,000 advance; retail; Feminist, mainstream, and contemporary themes on women showing creative slant on nonfiction, technical how-to approach to books.

Perspective Press: PO Box 90318, Indianapolis, IN 46290-0318; 317-872-3055; Pat Johnston, Publisher; est: 1982; 200 mss/yr; 4 titles/yr; 5-15%/retail; Focus on adults seeking latest input on fertility decisions and adoptive/foster parenting issues.

Peterson's: PO Box 2123, Princeton, NJ 08543-2123; 800-338-3282; Carole Cushmore, Publishing; est: 1966; 250 mss/yr; 55-75 titles/yr; 10-12%/retail; High profile direct-mail publisher in self-help business, careers, education, and family and child guidance books. Accepts consumer directories.

Pfeiffer & Company: 8517 Production Avenue, San Diego, CA 92121; 619-578-2042; 619-578-5900; JoAnn Padgett, Managing Editor; est: 1968; 80 titles/yr; 10%/retail; Paperback business themes in human resource development, group-oriented and management education materials, classroom teacher guides, and practical how-to manuals.

Piccadilly Books: PO Box 25203, Colorado Springs, CO 80936-5203; 719-548-1844; Bruce Fife, Publisher; est: 1985; 120 mss/yr; 3-8 titles/yr; 5-10%/retail; Smaller self-help and practical books on performing arts, business, humor, business, and building careers in comedy and entertainment.

Prep Publishing: 1110 1/2 Hay Street, Fayetteville, NC 28305; 910-483-6611; Anne McKinney, Managing Editor; 500 mss/yr; 10 titles/yr; 6-17%/retail; Spritual and secular self-help approach to money, finance, psychology, career advice, appealing to widespread early twenties audience.

Presidio Press: 505B San Martin Drive, Suite 300, Novato, CA 94945-1340; 415-898-0383; 415-898-1081; E.J. McCarthy, Executive Editor; est: 1974; 1,000 mss/yr; 24 titles/yr; 15-20%/net; Leading publisher in military affairs and military history of true crime, realistic portrayals, psychological autopsies of military battles, and autobiographies of military heroes.

Pride Publications: PO Box 148, Radnor, OH 43066-0148; 603-225-5651; 603-225-5651; pridepblsh@aol.com; Keystone books, routing; est: 1989; 75 mss/ yr; 5 titles/yr; 10-15%/wholesale; All genres in how-to, self-help on subjects of personal growth, development, parenting, childcare, aging.

Prima Publishing: PO Box 1260, Rocklin, CA 95677-1260; 916-768-0426; Jennifer Bayse-Sander, Senior Acquisitions Editor; 750 mss/yr; 300 titles/yr; 15-20%/wholesale; Enterprising publisher drawing bookseller attention lately in original, authoritative books on health, psychology, business, and covering most addiction-recovery topics.

Prometheus Books: 59 John Glenn Drive, Buffalo, NY 14228; 716-837-2475; Steven Mitchell, Editorial Director; est: 1969; 2,000 mss/yr; 25-30 titles/yr; Leading small press featuring works in politics, health, fitness, science, paranormal, sexuality, history, religion, and general trade.

QED Press: 155 Cypress Street, Fort Bragg, CA 95437; 707-964-9520; qed-press@mcn.org; John Fremont, Senior Editor; 2,000 mss/yr; 10 titles/yr; 7-15% /retail; Seeking books on aging, health process, careers for elders, investments, and psychology self-help on later-year development.

Quest Books: PO Box 270, Wheaton, IL 60189; 708-665-5791; 708-665-0130; questbooks@aol.com; Brenda Rosen, Executive Editor; 150 mss/yr; 12-15 titles/ yr; 10-12%/retail; Small tradebook press featuring metaphysical, spiritual, religion, psychology, health and medicine.

Random House: 201 East 50th Street, New York, NY 10022; 212-751-2600; 3,000 mss/yr; 120 titles/yr; Inquire about their specific imprints (e.g., Alfred A. Knopf, Ballantine, Crown, Fawcett, Vintage) on areas covering psychology, nature, sports. May require agent inquiry.

Resource Publications, Inc.: 160 E. Virginia Street, Suite 290, San Jose, CA 95112-5876; 408-287-8748; kenneth856@aol.com; Kenneth E. Guentert, Editorial Director; est: 1973; 200 mss/yr; 14 titles/yr; 8%/retail; Books providing practical, how-to suggestions in counseling, pastoral guidance, education, and secular direction on drug abuse prevention, domestic assault, and other social problems.

Rising Tide Press: 5 Kivy Street, Huntington Station, NY 11746-2020; 516-427-1289; rtpress@aol.com; Alice Frier, Senior Editor; est: 1991; 150 mss/yr; 10-20 titles/yr; 10-15%/wholesale; Concentrates on lesbian issues, lives, and self-help direction on emotional, medical, and personal adjustment.

St. Martin's Press: 175 5th Avenue, New York, NY 10010; 212-420-9314; 212-674-5151; Keith Kahla, Editor; est: 1952; 200 mss/yr; 10%/retail; Strongly promotes first-time authors or on prestigious topics of self-help, military history, true crime, business.

Harold Shaw Publishers: 388 Gunderson Drive, PO Box 567, Wheaton, IL 60189; 708-665-6700; Joan Guest, Managing Editor; est: 1967; 4,000 mss/yr; 38 titles/yr; 5-10%/retail; General nonfiction with unusual consumer twist ranging from how-to's on marriage, family, parenting, spiritual growth, Bible study and where obvious marketing angle promises large presales.

Sibyl Publications: 123 NE Third Avenue, #502, Portland, OR 97232; 503-231-7492; 503-231-6519; Miriam Selby, Publisher; 4-6 titles/yr; $500-1,000 advance; 10-15%/wholesale; Target readership is midlife women, ages 36-60, seeking answers in spirituality, mythology, psychology, women's studies, with compelling theme for impulse purchasers.

Sourcebooks, Inc.: PO Box 313, Naperville, IL 60566; 708-961-2168; 708-961-3900; Todd Stocke, Associate Editor; est: 1987; 35 titles/yr; 6-15%/whoesale; Self-help, short guidebooks on parenting, childcare, psychology, motivation–all with electrifying titles and innovative ideas for small business owners, entrepreneurs, and students.

The Speech Bin, Inc.: 1965 25th Avenue, Vero Beach, FL 32960-3062; 407-770-0007; Jan Binney, Senior Editor; est: 1984; 500 mss/yr; 10-20 titles/yr; Increasingly visible publisher with speciality in self-help, consumer books on communication disorders, illustrated juvenile books for handicapped persons, and health-related, sold to special educators, parents, teachers, caregivers.

Spinsters Ink: 32 E. First Street, #330, Duluth, MN 55802; 218-727-3119; 218-727-3222; spinsters@aol.com;http.//www.lesbian.org/spinsters-ink. Jamie Snyder, Editor; est: 1978; 200 mss/yr; 6 titles/yr; 7-11%/retail; Feminist and lesbian proactive social books with self-help guides on emotional changes, written by and for women.

Starburst Publishers: PO Box 4123, Lancaster, PA 17604; 717-293-0939; Ellen Hake, Editorial Director; est: 1982; 1,000 mss/yr; 10-15 titles/yr; 6-15%/retail; General how-to from Christian perspective sold to religious lay marketplace on health, medicine, self-help, money, and finance.

Sterling Publishing: 387 Park Avenue South, New York, NY 10016; 212-213-2495; 212-532-7160; Sheila Anne Barry, Acquisitions Manager; est: 1949; Focuses on alternative lifestyle in topics ranging from ghosts to health with how-to orientation.

Stillpoint Publishing: PO Box 640, Walpole, NH 03608; 603-756-9282; 603-756-9281; Dorothy Seymour, Senior Editor; 500 mss/yr; 8-10 titles/yr; Seeking theme-supported how-to and helping guides on personal growth, spiritual development, business, work and community, overall focusing on global well-being.

Success Publishing: PO Box 30965, Palm Beach Gardens, FL 33420; 407-775-1693; 407-626-4643; Robin Garretson, Submission Manager; est: 1982; 200 mss/

yr; 6 titles/yr; 7%/retail; Target audience is housewives, hobbyists, and small business owners looking for how-to subjects on business, economics, money, and finance.

Sulzburger & Graham Publishing, Ltd.: 165 West 91st Street, New York, NY 10024; Neil Blond, Publisher; 100 mss/yr; 35 titles/yr; $100-200 advance; 15%/wholesale; Many self-help imprints (e.g., Human Services Institute) focusing on business, career, child guidance, parenting, computers, health, travel, psychology.

The Summit Publishing Group: One Arlington Center, 112 E. Copeland, 5th floor, Arlington, TX 76011; Mike Towle, Managing Edtior; 25-30 titles/yr; up to $15,000 advance; 5-20%/wholesale; High profile titles and strong market books for national distribution covering health, medicine, money, finance, psychology, military, sports, women's issues.

Swan-Raven & Company: PO Box 726, Newberg, OR 97132; 503-538-8485; 503-538-0264; Amy Owen, Editor; 25 mss/yr; 6 titles/yr; 5-12%/wholesale; Small press articulating new age, future speculation, health, philosophy, self-help, and women's issues.

Taylor Publishing Company: 1550 W. Mockingbird Lane, Dallas, TX 75235; 214-819-8580; 214-819-8560; http://www.taylorpub.com; Crystal Blackburn, Editor; est: 1981; 1,000 mss/yr; 30 titles/yr; Taylor's expanding list now includes subjects on gardening, parenting, health, personal improvement, and lifestyle.

Third-Side Press, Inc.: 2250 W. Farragut, Chicago, IL 60625; http://www.small-media.com; Midge Stocker, Publisher; 4-5 titles; 6%/retail; Contemporary self-help and business highlighting women, feminism, lesbianism, women's health issues.

Thunder's Mouth Press: 632 Broadway, 7th Floor, New York, NY 10012; 212-780-0380; Neil Ortenberg, Publisher; est: 1982; 1,000 mss/yr; 15-20 titles/yr; $15,000 advance; 5-10%/retail; Generally covers popular culture subjects from self-help and psychology to politics and biography.

Todd Publications: 18 N. Greenbush Road, West Nyack, NY 10994; 914-358-6213; toddpub@aol.com; Barry Klein, President; 5 titles/yr; 5-15%/wholesale; Rapidly growing publisher promoting self-help in ethnic, health, medicine, psychology, money, finance topics.

Trilogy Books: 50 S. Delacey Avenue, Suite 201, Pasadena, CA 91105; 818-440-0669; Marge Wood, Publisher; 4 titles/yr; 4-10%/retail; Mainstreamed readers of feminism, women's studies, history, and topics overlapping academic and trade nonfiction markets.

Triumph Books: 333 Glen Head Road, Old Brookville, NY 11545; 818-585-9441; 818-440-0669; 72274,44@compuserve.com; Patricia A. Kossman, Executive Editor; 75 titles/yr; $2,500-7,500 advance; 7-15%/retail; Building line of inspirational, spiritual books grounded in self-help on psychology, women's issues, and theology.

Tudor Publishers: PO Box 38366, Greensboro, NC 27438; 910-282-5907; Pam Cox, Senior Editor; 400 mss/yr; 4-6 titles/yr; 10%/wholesale; Paperback trade publisher of biography, psychology, self-help, child guidance, parenting, nutrition, history, sports, and cooking.

Valley of the Sun Publishing: PO Box 38, Malibu, CA 90265; Richard Sutphen, Publisher; 2,000 mss/yr; 6 titles/yr; $1,500-2,000 advance; Increasing shopping line of new age, UFO, self-help, metaphysical, personal growth.

Viking Studio Books: 375 Hudson Street, New York, NY 10014; 212-366-2191; Michael Fragnito, Publisher; 200 mss/yr; 35-40 titles/yr; Imprint of Penguin USA books with commercial nonfiction line for health, medicine, military, war, self-help, recovery, and addiction.

Villard Books: 201 E. 50th Street, New York, NY 10022; 212-572-2780; Craig Nelson, Editor-in-Chief; est: 1983; 55-60 titles/yr; Imprint of Random House seeking strongly marketable nonfiction trade in all areas with prolific author credentials. Contact through literary agents only.

Walker & Company: 435 Hudson Street, New York, NY 10014; 212-727-0984; 212-727-8300; Michael Seidman, Editor; est: 1959; 4,500 mss/yr; 100 titles/yr; $1,000-3,000 advance; 6-12%/retail; Biography, business, true crime, psychology, self-help, and several practical books aimed for mainstream readership.

Samuel Weiser, Inc.: PO Box 612, York Beach, ME 03910-0612; 207-363-5799; 207-363-4393; Eliot Stearns, Editor; est: 1956; 200 mss/yr; 18-20 titles/yr; $500 advance; 10%/wholesale; Specialist publisher in oriental philosophy, esoterica, metaphysics, self-help in psychology and astrology, with proof of author expertise.

Westport Publishers, Inc.: 1102 Grand, 23rd Floor, Kansas City, MO 64106; 816-842-8188; 816-842-8111; Paul Temme, Publisher; est: 1982; 125 mss/yr; 5-12 titles/yr; Host of modern genres from parenting and childcare to personal growth and women's studies from experts in field.

Whitford Press: 77 Lower Valley Road, Atglen, PA 19310; 610-593-1777; Ellen Taylor, Managing Editor; est: 1985; 400-500 mss/yr; 1-3 titles/yr; wholesale; New age publisher expanding metaphysical line to paranormal phenomena, progressive transpersonal material, and astrology.

Wilshire Book Company: 12015 Sherman Road, North Hollywood, CA 91605; 818-765-2922; 818-765-8579; Melvin Powers, Publisher; est: 1947; 3,000 mss/yr; 50 titles/yr; Commercial high profile trade line of psychology, success, self-help books promising large sales.

Woodbridge Press: PO Box 209, Santa Barbara, CA 93102; 805-965-7039; Howard Weeks, Editor; est: 1971; 300 mss/yr; 4-5 titles/yr; 10-15%/wholesale; Self-help manuals on eating (vegetarian), psychology and recovery, gardening, and health.

Zoland Books, Inc.: 384 Huron Avenue, Cambridge, MA 02138; 617-661-4998; 617-864-6252; Roland Pease Jr., Publisher; est: 1987; 400 mss/yr; 8-12 titles/yr;

7%/retail; Subjects include thought-provoking trades in arts, women's issues, self-help healing, and personal growth.

Zondervan Publishing House: 5300 Patterson Avenue SE, Grand Rapids, MI 49530-0002; 616-698-6900; Editorial Coordinator; est: 1931; 3,000 mss/yr; 130 titles/yr; 12%/retail; Large religious publisher for academic and trade nonfiction spanning humanities (preaching, counseling, self-help, worship) and how-to guides in biblical reference.

POPULAR MAGAZINE PUBLISHERS

Next are magazine resources. The following resources are only paying magazines. They run the gamut from sports to animal training. Each entry follows a sequence of information completed based on the replies from each magazine editor or publisher. Entirely completed entries include the following:

Name of Magazine: address; city, state, zip code; fax number; phone number; e-mail or URL (web page) address; editor; date established; number of manuscripts submitted per year (mss/yr.); number of features published per year (features/yr.); number of words in manuscripts requested (words); orientation and subject of magazine with tips for authors and properties needed.

Animals

AKC Gazette: Mark Roland, Features Editor; 51 Madison Ave, 19th Floor, New York, NY 10010; 212-696-8299;212-696-8331; circ: 55,000; monthly; pays $200-$300; 1,000-2,500 words; byline; est: 1889; Official outlet for sport of purebred dogs to provide secrets to great showmanship with articles on veterinary medicine, behavior, grooming, nutrition, and professional training and obedience.

Animals: Joni Praded, Editor; 350 S. Huntington Ave, Boston, MA 02130; 617-522-4885;617-522-7400; circ: 100,000; bimonthly; pays $350; 2,200 words; 8 mss/yr; byline; est: 1868; Well-researched facts combined with lively feature stories on animal behavior, lifestyle, and interaction with nature.

Animal's Agenda: KW Stallwood, Editor; PO Box 25881, Baltimore, MD 21224; 410-675-0066; 410-675-4566; circ: 20,000; bimonthly; pays $100; 1,000-3,000 words; 1-10 mss/yr; byline; est: 1979; Practical holistic approach and investigative reporting on human treatment toward animals, including societal, political, and agricultural perspectives.

Appaloosa Journal: A.J. Mangum, Editor; 5070 Hwy, 8 West, Box 8403, Moscow, ID 83843; 208-882-8150; 208-882-5578; circ: 14,000 monthly; pays

$100-$400; 400-3,000 words; 4-6 mss/yr.; byline; est: 1946; Designed to meet needs of the Appaloosa horse club emphasizing trends in breeding, training, animal health, and marketing.

Arabian Horse Express: Kathleen Gallagher, Editor; 512 Green Bay Rd, Ste. 302, Kenilworth, IL 60043-1073; 708-256-5898; 800-533-9734; circ: 10,000; monthly; byline; Newsmagazine for Arabian horse owners and enthusiasts on sportsmanship, training, breeding, and rapport.

Audubon: Michael Robbins, Editor; 700 Broadway, New York, NY 10003; bimonthly; pays $800-$4,000; 1,500-4,000 words; 85 features/yr; byline; Perspectives on wildlife, environment, ecology, stories of people, places affecting humans and nature in conflict.

Bird Talk: Kathleen Etchetare, Editor; 3 Burroughs, Irvine, CA 92718; 714-855-3045; 714-855-8822; circ:160,000; monthly; pays $.10-$.15/word; 500-3,000 words; 150 mss/yr; byline; Targeted to bird lovers focusing on nutrition, medical, training, and breeding guidance including technical and human interest materials.

Cat Fancy: Jane Calloway, Managing Editor; PO Box 605, Mission Viejo, CA 92690; 714-855-3045; 714-855-8822; circ: 303,000; monthly; pays $25-$450; 400-2,000 words; byline; est: 1945; Cat lovers almanac delving into all aspects of cat care from nutrition and choosing correct cat to breed profiles, training, and product reviews.

Cats Magazine: Tracey Copeland, Features Editor, PO Box 290037; Port Orange, FL 32129-0037; 904-788-2710; 904-788-2770; catsmag@aol.com; circ: 10,500; monthly; pays $35-$400; 500-3,000 words; 5-7 mss/yr; byline; est:1965; Authoritative periodical for feline enthusiasts, providing latest facts for breeders and exhibitors on a broad range from veterinarian and behavior to book reviews.

Chronicle of the Horse: Nancy Comer, Editor; PO Box 46, Middleburg, VA 22117-0046; 703-687-3937; 703-687-6341; circ: 23,000; weekly; pays $25-$200; 300-1,225 words; 300 mss/yr; byline; est: 1937; Historical and nostalgic overview of horsemanship profiling major competitions, breeding, training, racing, riding, and official business for organizations governing these subspecialties.

Dog Fancy: Kim Campbell Thornton, Editor; PO Box 6050, Mission Viejo, CA 92690; 714-855-3045; 714-855-8822; circ: 290,000 monthly; varies; 750-3,000 words; 36 mss/yr; byline; est: 1970; For serious dog owners seeking highlights of breeding, care, training of purebreds and mixed breeds, with focus on pet care and grooming.

Dog World: Donna Marcel, editor; 29 N Wacker Drive, Chicago IL 60606-3298; 312-726-4103; 312-726-4340; dogworld3@aol.com; circ: 63,000; monthly; negotiable; 10 mss/issue; byline; est: 1916; Dog enthusiast's bible for contemporary styles and trends in industry, from conformation and obedience exhibition, grooming, kennel operations, veterinarians, and hobby breeding. Attracts longtime dog owners reading on healthcare, dog behavior.

Equine Market: Midge Koontz, Editor, 111 Shore Dr., Hinsdale, IL 60521; 708-887-1958; 708-887-7722; circ: 5,000; monthly; pays $25; 500-3,000 words; 70 mss/yr; byline; est: 1970; For sophisticated equestrian riders reporting technical and travel tips along with personal experience on training, product usage, and leisure.

Equus: Laurie Prinz, Managing Editor; 656 Quince Orchard Rd., Gaithersburg, MD 20878-1409; 301-990-9015; 301-977-3900; circ: 132,000; monthly; byline; For horse owners seeking latest information on horse care and performance. Articles cover veterinary topics, stable management, behavioral training, and riding.

Greyhound Review: Tim Horan, Editor; PO Box 543, Abilene, KS 67410; 913-263-4689; 913-263-4660; circ: 6,000; monthly; pays $100-$150; 1,000-10,000 words; 24 mss/yr; byline; est: 1911; How-to personal experience exploring racetrack and medical discoveries on breeding, training, and raising greyhounds.

Horse and Horseman: Claudia Dane, Managing Editor; 34249 Camino Capistrano, Capistrano Beach, CA 92624-1156; 714-240-8680; 714-493-2101; circ: 89,380; monthly; byline; Designed for people who ride, own, train, and breed popular breeds of horses. Highlights tips on how-to of training, caring, feeding, and riding for pleasure and competition.

Horse Illustrated: Audrey Pavia, Editor; PO Box 6050, Mission Viejo, CA 92690-6050; 714-855-3045; 714-855-8822; circ: 176,353; monthly; pays $50-$300; 1,000-2,500 words; 100 mss/yr; byline; est: 1976; Features stories, articles on riding both English and Western, all breeds, and covers owner care, health, performance, conditioning, feeding, and showing.

Horseplay: Lisa Kiser, Editor; 11 Park Avenue, Gaithersburg, MD 20877-2915; 301-840-5722; 301-840-1866; circ: 43,500; monthly; pays $.10/word; 2,500 words or less; byline; Tailored for competitive and recreational English-style horseback riders, focused on riding, training, breeding, health, nutrition, conditioning, equipment, news, and events.

I Love Cats: Lisa Sheets, Editor; 950 Third Avenue, 16th Floor, New York, NY 10022-2705; 212-888-8420; 212-888-1855; circ: 180,500; bimonthly; pays $40-$250; 100-1,000 words; 200 mss/yr; byline; est: 1989; News and information for cat owners focusing on nutrition, veterinary advice, homeopathic remedies, personal stories, and behavior training.

Monkey Matters: Randy Helm, Editor; PO Box 62, Moraga, CA 94556; 510-274-6210; circ: 2,000; bimonthly; pays $5; 500-2,500 words; 24 mss/yr; byline; est: 1995; Inspirational tabloid covering natural habitat and behavior of primates, emphasizing personal stories, insights, and applied technical methods for raising, training, and programs helping human beings.

Mushing: Diane Herrmann, Editor; PO Box 149, Ester, AK 99725-0149; 907-479-0454; 907-479-0454; circ: 6,000; bimonthly; pays $50-$250; 500-3,000 words; byline; est: 1987; Focuses on all aspects of dog-driving activities including departments in health, training, personality, historical, and general breeding.

Paint Horse Journal: Darrell Dodds, Editor; PO Box 961023, Fort Worth, TX 76161-0023; 817-439-3484; 817-439-3400; circ: 20,850; monthly; pays $24-$40; 4-5 mss/yr; byline; est: 1966; Edited for serious amateur horsemen to promote the paint horse industry, focusing on health, training, breeding, and showing of horses.

Associations

Elks Magazine: Judith L Keogh, Editor; 425 W. Diversey, Chicago, IL 60614-6196; 312-528-4500; elksmag@aol.com; http://www.elksmag.com; circ: 1 million; 10 times/yr; pays $150+; 3,000 words; 2-3 mss/yr; byline; est: 1922; Edited for general Elks membership and their families, emphasizing health, travel, retirement planning, local news, and emotional growth.

Kiwanis: Chuck Jonak, Editor; 3636 Woodview Trace, Indianapolis, IN 46268-3196; 317-879-0204; 317-875-8755; circ: 279,666; 10 times/yr; pays $500-$1,000; 2,200-2,600 words; 40 features/yr; byline; est: 1917; Attention grabbing stories with investigative flaire for personal and community growth tailored for members of Kiwanians clubs.

The Optimist: Dennis R. Osterwisch, Editor; 4494 Lindell Blvd., St. Louis, MO 63108-2404; 314-371-6006; 314-371-6000; dlockoi@aol.com; circ: 155,000; 6 times/yr; pays $75-$400; 500-1,000 words; 15-20 features/yr; byline; est: 1919; Official publication of Optimist International, providing news and information on motivation, growth, and life-building stories.

The Rotarian: Charles Pratt, Managing Editor; 1560 Sherman Ave., Evanston, IL 60201-3698; 708-866-9732; 708-866-3000; 75457.3577@compuserve.com; http://www.rotary.org; circ: 524,395; monthly; pays $300-$1,000; 1,200-1,500 words; 50-75 features/yr; byline; est: 1911; General interest articles on medicine, sports, business, management, and international affairs appealing to members of Rotary Club.

Scouting: Jon C. Halter, Editor; 1325 W. Walnut Hill Lane, Irving, TX 75015-2079; 214-580-2079; 214-580-2367; 103064.3363@compuserve.com; circ: 900,000; bimonthly; pays $200-$800; 500-1,000 words; 60 mss/yr; byline; est: 1913; Directed to volunteer adult Club, Scout, and Explorer leaders focused on specific programs, educational functions, leadership, nature, travel, health and psychology, family relationships, and issues on American heritage.

The Toastmaster: Suzanne Frey, Editor; PO Box 9052, Mission Viejo, CA 92690-7052; 714-858-1207; 714-858-8255; circ: 170,000; monthly; pays $75-250; 1,000-2,500; 50 mss/yr; byline; est: 1932; Highlights educational and how-to articles about public speaking, communications, and leadership consistent with goals of Toastmasters Organizations.

VFW Magazine: Rich Kolb, Editor; 406 W. 34th St., Kansas City, MO 64111; 816-968-1169; 816-756-3390; circ: 2.1 million; monthly; pays $500 max; 1,500 words; 25-30 mss/yr; byline; Nostalgic and news magazine highlighting veteran's affairs in military history, patriotism, defense, and current events, largely for those serving in armed forces overseas during World War II through Haiti.

Astrology and New Age

FATE: Editor; PO Box 64383, St. Paul, MN 55164-0383; 612-291-1908; monthly; pays $.10/word; 2,000-4,000 words; byline; est: 1901; Articles delve into science and interesting accounts of psychic and mystical phenomena including cryptozoology, parapsychology, spiritual healing, flying saucers, and new discoveries of ancient civilizations.

Gnosis: Richard Smoley, Editor; PO Box 14217, San Francisco, CA 94114; 415-255-0400; smoley@well.com; circ: 16,000; quarterly; pays $50-$200; 1,000-5,000 words; 32 mss/yr; byline; est: 1985; Thematic magazine focusing on Western esoteric spirituality integrating Judaism, Christianity, Islam, and Paganism, including mystical and occult traditions.

New Age Journal: Lisa Horvitz, Editor; 42 Pleasant St., Watertown, MA 02127; 617-926-5021; swamiv@aol.com; bimonthly; pays $50-$2,500; 500-4,000 words; 60-80 mss/yr; byline; Reaches college-educated 25 to 45 year olds looking for reconciliation of spiritual with personal values in humanitarian outlook on life, with issues on plants, behavior, high-tech, and inspiration.

New Frontier: Swami Virato, Editor; PO Box 17397, Asheville, NC 28806-2724; swamiv.aol; circ: 60,000; bimonthly; pays $50; 1,500-4,000 words; 15 mss/yr; byline; est: 1980; Focuses on transformation of human consciousness dealing with ecology, spirituality, self-help, metaphysics, Eastern philosophy, cosmology, altered states, and health and natural foods.

Business

Executive Female: Dorian Burden, Editor; 30 Irving Place, 5th Floor, New York, NY 10003; 212-477-8215; 212-477-2200; nafe@nafe.com; http://www.nafe.com; circ: 192,000; bimonthly; pays $.50/word; 800-2,000 words; byline; est: 1975; Concentrates on career and financial management for managerial women with topics ranging from ethics to stress including romance, economics, and office relationships.

Family PC: JoAnn Hirschel, Managing Editor; 244 Main Street, Northampton, MA 01060; 413-582-9070; 413-582-9200; familypc@aol.com; circ: 200,000; monthly; byline; Provides timely and entertaining articles on technology, products, group activities, and accessories for computer literate families.

New Writer's Magazine: George J. Haborak, Editor; PO Box 5976, Sarasota, FL 34277; 941-953-7903; 941-953-7903; newriters@aol.com; circ: 5,000; bimonthly; pays $15-$40; 750-800 words; 5 features/yr; byline; est: 1986; Magazine is a publication for aspiring writers and professionals. It serves as a meeting place where all writers freely exchange thoughts, ideas, backgrounds, and work samples, plus it keeps writers informed on market trends. Guidelines available.

Working Woman: Lynn Povich, Editor; 230 Park Avenue, New York, NY 10169-0005; 212-599-4763; 212-551-9500; wwedit@womweb.com; circ: 764,594; monthly; byline; est: 1991; Reports stirring trends and career shifts on family, lifestyle, romance, office politics, and entrepreneurship.

Your Money: Dennis Fertig, Editor; 5705 N. Lincoln Ave., Chicago, IL 60659; 312-275-3590; circ: 500,000; bimonthly; pays $.50/word; 1,500-2,500 words; 25 mss/yr; byline; est: 1979; Investment tabloid outlining opportunities and solutions to today's economic questions for upscale clients in high salary bracket, with research-based versus first-person success stories.

Career and College

The Black Collegian: Sonya Stenson, Editor; 140 Carondelet Street, New Orleans, LA 70130; 504-523-0271; 504-523-0154; circ: 121,000; semi-annual; pays $100-$500; 500-1,500 words; 40 mss/yr; byline; est: 1970; Designed as guide for career and self-development for Black American college seniors and young professionals emphasizing job-hunting tips, review sources, financial aid, self-esteem builders, investigations of racial conditions affecting progress.

Career Focus: Neoshia Michelle Paige, Editor; 250 Mark Twain Tower, 106 W. 11th St., Kansas City, MO 64105; 516-273-8936; 516-221-4404; circ: 250,000; monthly; pays $150-$400; 750-2,000 words; byline; est: 1988; Provides inspirational direction for Hispanics and Afro-Americans, ages 21-40, with educational, vocational, and career options focused on success profile stories, advancement opportunities, and solutions to societal roadblocks.

Careers & Colleges: June Rogoznica, Editor; 989 Avenue of the Americas, Sixth Floor, New York, NY 10018; 212-967-2531; 212-563-4688; circ: 18,000; semi-annual; pays $150 minimum; 600-1,500 words; 36-52 mss/yr; byline; est: 1980; Provides update facts for high school juniors and seniors who plan to pursue advanced degrees or begin their careers. Includes job and interview tips, career profiles, and advice for choosing and applying to college.

Direct Aim: Neoshia Michelle Paige, Editor; 106 W. 11th Street, #250, Kansas City, MO 64105-1806; 816-221-1112; 816-221-4404; circ: 500,000; quarterly; pays $150-$400; 750-2,000 words; byline; Written for Black and Hispanic students in colleges, universities, junior colleges, and vocational school on establishing careers and entering the hectic world, featuring individual profiles, celebrities, and goals of persistence.

For Seniors Only: Meredith Fahn, Features Editor; 339 N. Main Street, New City, NY 10956-4300; 914-634-9423; 914-638-0333; circ: 350,000; semi-annual; byline; Mainstream magazine for high-school seniors dealing with methods for succeeding in college, summer job opportunties, preparing resumes, information on scholarships, military opportunities, and tips for smooth life transitions.

Childcare and Families

Adoptive Families: Linda Lynch, Editor; 3333 Highway 100 N., Minneapolis, MN 55422; 612-535-7808; 612-535-4829; circ: 25,000; bimonthly; byline; Material includes in-depth stories and features on issues affecting adoptive parents including waiting games, family library, single parents, birth parents, living with diversity, and personal stories.

All About Kids: Earladeen Badger, Editor; 1077 Celestial Street, #101, Cincinnati, OH 45202-1629; 513-684-0507; 513-684-0501; circ: 55,000; monthly; byline; Reinforces the mental health of mothers by focusing on health and well-being of newborns and expectant experience. Highlights nutrition, beauty tips, maternity and infant status, and personal relationships.

American Baby: Judith Nolte, Editor; 249 W. 17th Street, New York, NY 10011-5300; 212-463-6413; 212-645-0067; circ: 1 million; monthly; pays $350-$1,000; 1,000-2,000 words; 96 features/yr; byline; How-to facts and information for expectant parents from experts and reassuring personal stories.

At Home: Stewart McClure, Editor; 914 S. Santa Fe Avenue #297, Vista, CA 92084; 619-598-9285; 619-598-9260; circ: 300; bimonthly; byline; Boosts mothers enthusiasm to be full-time mothers focusing on stay-at-home industry, time management, home organization, fitness, craft ideas, marriage, and family.

Atlanta Parent: Peggy Middendorf, Editor; 4330 Georgetown Square II, Suite #506, Atlanta, GA 30338; 770-454-7699; 770-454-7699; http:/www.family.com; circ: 65,000; 4 times/yr; pays $15-$25 features; 600-1,200 words; 75 mss/yr; byline; Parents and children ages birth through fourteen on family life, child care, public and private schools, motherhood, and drug abuse.

Baby Talk: Talley Sue Hohlfeld, Managing Editor; 5 W. 43rd Street, New York, NY 10036-7406; 212-840-0019; 212-840-4200; circ: 1 million; monthly; byline; Expectant and new parents looking for awareness of first year of life. Columns cover health, pregnancy tips, birth, childcare, nutrition, marriage, and finance.

Bay Area Parent Magazine: Lynn Berardo, Editor; 401 "A" Alberto Way, Los Gatos, CA 95032-5404; 408-356-4903; 408-358-1414; bap@ual.com; circ: 60,000; monthly; pays $.06/word; 600-1,000 words; 60-70 mss/yr; byline; Parents of children, newborns to teens, stressing childrearing, development, education, child-related products and publications, and health/psychological advice for growing families.

Black Child: Candy Mills, Editor; 2870 Peachtree Road, NW #264, Atlanta, GA 30305; 404-364-9965; 404-364-9690; circ: 50,000; bimonthly; pays $35-$50; 800 words; byline; est: 1995; Parenting or childcare theme limited to black families on news, events, success stories, research, and race relations.

Child of Color: Candy Mills, Editor; 2870 Peachtree Road, NW #264, Atlanta, GA 30305; 404-364-9965; 404-364-9690; circ: 5,000; quarterly; 800 words;

byline; est: 1996; Magazine for parenting issues affecting whites, Asians, Latinos, Native Americans, multi-ethnic children, and societal and family problems faced.

Child Magazine: Miriam Arond, Articles Editor; 110 Fifth Avenue, New York, NY 10011-5699; 212-463-1383; 212-463-1000; childmag@aol.com; circ: 700,000; monthly; 1,800-2,000 words; 40 features/yr; byline; est: 1986; Covers developmental stages, parenting, siblinghood, marriages and divorce, and family lifestyles.

Christian Parenting Today: Brad Lewis, Editor; 4050 Lee Vance View, Colorado Springs, CO 80936-3663; 719-535-0172; 719-531-7776; circ: 250,000; bimonthly; pays $.15-$.25/word; 750-2,000 words; 50 mss/yr; byline; est: 1988; Edited for contemporary family addressing isssues of child raising, health, mental development, development, and self-esteem, all from Christian or biblical perspective.

Exceptional Parent: Stanley Klein, Editor; 209 Harvard St., Suite 303, Brookline, MA 02146; 617-730-8742; 617-730-5800; circ: 50,000; monthly; pays $25 max; 50 mss/yr; byline; est: 1971; Prepared for parents, educators, and health professionals working with disabled children. Content on curricula, development, legislation, behavior management, literature reviews.

Expecting: Maija Johnson, Editor; 685 Third Avenue, 29th Floor, New York, NY 10017-4024; 212-867-4583; 212-878-8700; circ: 1 million; quarterly; byline; Articles on latest subjects of concern for pregnant women consisting of carefully researched articles on health, maternity, fashions, proper mental health, and family balance.

The Family: Theresa Frances Myers, Editor; 50 St. Paul's Avenue, Boston, MA 02130; 617-541-9805; 617-522-8911; monthly; byline; Designed to respond to modern Catholic family issues, featuring talk on personal and family problems through spiritual outlook.

Family: Stacy Brassington, Editor; 169 Lexington Avenue, New York, NY 10016; 212-779-3080; 212-545-9740; circ: 558,934; monthly; byline; Provides military wives with comprehensive and informative updates on parenting, travel, issues impacting military families, book reviews, and childcare.

Family Circle: Nancy Clark, Deputy Editor; 110 Fifth Avenue, New York, NY 10011; 212-463-1808; 212-463-1000; circ: 5 million; 17 issues/yr; pays $1/word; 1,000-2,500 words; 200 features/yr; byline; Tabloid profiles family and personal relationships, self-improvement, nutrition, and community activities.

Family Fun: Clare Ellis, Editor; 244 Main St., Northampton, MA 01060; circ: 675,000; 10 times/yr; pays $.50/word; 75-3,000 words; 100+ mss/yr; byline; est: 1991; Provides variety of family activities and parenting insights for parents with kids ages 3-12, covering relationships and traditions, great ideas, disciplinary startegies, and fiction stories.

Family Life: Wendy Israel, Managing Editor; 1633 Broadway, 41st Floor, New York, NY 10019; 212-489-4561; 212-767-4918; familylife@aol.com; circ:

400,000; monthly; pays $1/word; byline; est: 1993; Written explicitly for parents of children ages 3 to 12 and focused on education, holidays, health, and role of parent in formative years.

Family Times: Alison Stooker Garber, Editor; 1900 Superfine Lane, Wilmington, DE 19802; 302-575-0933; 302-575-0935; family@family.com; circ: 50,000; monthly; pays $30 min; 350-1,200 words; 60 mss/yr; byline; est: 1990; Dedicated to parents and caregivers living in Eastern region of United States, filled with parenting advice, activity ideas, and family planning strategies.

Healthy Kids: Judith Nolte, Editor; 249 W. 17th Street, New York, NY 10011; 212-463-6410; 212-463-6578; circ: 1 million; quarterly; pays $500-$1,000; 1,500-2,000 words; 30 mss/yr; byline; est: 1989; Targeting parents on children's health from birth to age 10, addressing physical, emotional, and behavioral changes with features on first-aid and development.

Interrace: Candy Mills, Editor; 2870 Peachtree Road, NW #264, Atlanta, GA 30305; 404-364-9965; 404-364-9690; bimonthly; complimentary copies; 800 words; byline; est: 1989; Parent of biracial children of other color from either an interracial marriage or through adoption. Discussed are social challenges, solutions, and support from experts and parents.

LA Parent: David Jamieson, Managing Editor; 443 E Irving Drive #D, Burbank, CA 91504; 818-841-4964; 818-846-0400; 73311.514@compuserve.com; circ: 100,000; monthly; pays $200-$300; 700-1,200 words; 60-75 mss/yr; byline; est: 1980; Written for parents in Southern California featuring education, health, social issues, and travel.

Mothering: Peggy O'Mara, Editor; PO Box 1690, Santa Fe, NM 87504; 505-986-8335; 505-984-8116; circ: 70,000; quarterly; byline; Inspirational articles on motherhood, parenthood, family life, emotional and medical experiences of maternity.

Parenting Magazine: Bonnie Monte, Medical/health Editor; 301 Howard, 17th Floor, San Francisco, CA 94105; 415-546-0578; 415-546-7575; raskinb@parenting.com; circ: 925,000; monthly; pays $500-$2,000; 1,700 words; 20-30 features/yr; byline; est: 1987; Offers progressive, upbeat look at medical, self-help, and fashionable parenting roles for readers ages 25 to 35.

Parents' Magazine: Catherine Winters, Medical/Health Editor; 685 Third Avenue, New York, NY 10017-4052; 212-867-4583; 212-878-8770; circ: 1 million; monthly; varies; 2,500 max; byline; est: 1926; Young women ages 18 to 34 with growing children looking for topics on family formation, daily needs, personal lifestyle, and romance, and departments on safety, development of child.

Raising Children: Trish Eaton, Editor; 6837 Nancy Ridge Drive #J, San Diego, CA 92121; 619-658-0957; 619-658-0098; circ: 60,000; bimonthly; byline; Features stories and departments for parents with children ages 7 to 17, on health and fitness, family, problems facing today's teens, and school-age children.

Sesame Street Parents: Susan Schneider, Executive Editor;1 Lincoln Plaza, 3rd Floor, New York, NY 10023; 212-875-6105; 212-875-6470; circ: 1 million; 10 times/yr; pays $750-$2,000; 1,500-2,000 words; 30-40 features/yr; byline; Needs child-development and how-to stories for aspiring parents of young children.

The Single Parent: Debbie Olefsky, Editor; 401 N. Michigan Avenue, 23rd Floor, Chicago, IL 60611-42676; 312-321-6869; 312-644-6610; circ: 70,000; quarterly; byline; Addresses widowed, separated, divorced, and never married parents raising children alone. Articles on single parenting, development, education, self-help, conerns regarding parental model including short fiction for children.

Smart Parenting: Keith Bellows, Editor; 100 Avenue of the Americas, 7th Floor, New York, NY 10013; 212-334-1260; 212-219-7436; circ: 50,000; byline; Source for upscale, affluent young parents featuring restaurants, calendar of events, insightful answers to daily problems, and synthesis of latest-breaking research news.

Successful Black Parenting: Marta Sanchez-Speer, Editor; PO Box 6359, Philadelphia, PA 19044; 215-537-7053; 215-537-7736; circ: 30,000; quarterly; byline; Portrays the unique patterns of black family life, offering insider tips on child development, parenting, and updated news for adults working with or raising black children.

Today's Family: Jan Mars, Editor; PO Box 46112, Eden Prairie, MN 55344; 612-975-5921; 612-975-2933; circ: 50,000; quarterly; pays $10-$50; 750-1,200 words; 50 mss/yr; byline; est: 1991; Directed to modern family with nontraditional values, including step families and single-parent families. Features reflect childcare, health, education, and social and physical development.

Twins Magazine: Jeane Cerne, Editor in Chief; 6740 Antioch #155, Merriam, KS 66204; 913-722-1767; 913-722-1090; http://www.twinsmagazine.com; circ: 55,000; bimonthly; pays $50; 1,000-3,000 words; 150 mss/yr; byline; est: 1984; Informs parents, caretakers about birthing and raising multiple children, with guidance on parenting, twin research, and steps enhancing family dynamics.

Working Mother Magazine: Linda Hamilton, Articles Editor; 230 Park Avenue, Room #747, New York, NY 10169-0005; 212-551-9757; 212-551-9500; childcare; circ: 925,000; monthly; pays $1.00/word; 2,000 words; 108-120 features/yr; byline; Strives to show how to balance family, career, romance, and personal needs for women ages 20 to 40.

Consumer

Atlantic Monthly: Jack Beatty, Editor; 745 Boylston Street, Boston, MI 02116-2603; 617-536-5925; 617-536-9500; atlanticm@aol.com;circ: 473,916; monthly; byline; News magazine focusing on political, economic, fine arts events and personalities in contemporary world. Focus is for educated reader.

Avenue: Laura Fisher, Features Editor; 950 3rd Avenue; New York, NY 10022; 212-758-7395; 212-758-9517; circ: 80,000; monthly; byline; For residents of affluent neighborhoods of metropolitan cities in United States focused on arts, food, fashion, style, and travel.

Homeworking: Georganne Fiumara, Editor; Mothers Home Network, Box 423, East Meadow, NY 11554; 516-997-0839; 516-997-7394; circ: 10,000; quarterly; pays $150; 300-1,000 words; 5-10 mss/yr; byline; Personal experience reporting of home success stories and opportunities geared for mothers electing to work at home rather than offices.

Income Opportunities: Eric Barnes, Editor; 1500 Broadway,; New York, NY 10036-4015; 212-302-8269; 212-642-0600; incomeed@aol.com; circ: 425,000; monthly; pays $200-$400; 600-2,500 words; 100 mss/yr; byline; est: 1956; Strategies for startup, advertising methods, advice for readers for success, stories of actual earnings, and steps for small operations advancement.

Income Plus Magazine: Donna Clapp, Editor; 73 Spring St., Ste. 303, New York, NY 10012; 212-925-3108; 212-925-3180; circ: 150,000; monthly; pays $200-$300; 900-2,000 words; 48 mss/yr; byline; est: 1989; Provides proven hands-on techniques for income-producing small owners and enterprising new careers featuring personality profiles on money, marketing, sales, and entrepreneurship.

Spare Time Magazine: Robert R. Warde, Editor; 5810 W. Oklahoma Ave, Milwaukee, WI 53219; 414-543-8110; circ: 300,000; 9 times/yr; pays $75-$300; 500-1,500 words; 24-54 mss/yr; byline; est: 1955; Publishes easy-to-understand blueprint information for anybody starting spare-time to save for travel, college, retirement, focused on simplicity, proven track records of success, and personality profiles.

Disability

Ability: Chet Cooper, Editor; 1682 Langley Avenue, Irvine, CA 92714; 714-250-7011; 714-854-8700; circ: 165,000; bimonthly; byline; Content focuses on issues, health, prevention, reporting effects of Americans with Disability Act, celebrity interviews, innovative technology, and personal strategies for healthy lifestyle.

Able: Angela Miele Melledy, Editor; PO Box 395, Old Bethpage, NY 11804; 516-938-1704; 516-939-2253; circ: 21,000; monthly; byline; Features expert commentary and insight regarding disabilities, calendar of events, columns on health, self-improvement in large print.

Accent on Living: Betty Garee, Editor; PO Box 700, Bloomington, IL 61702-0700; 309-378-4420; 309-378-2961; circ: 19,500; quarterly; pays $.10/word; 250-1,000 words; 50-60 mss/yr; byline; est: 1956; Authoritative forum for physically disabled readers, their families, and for professionals and laity working with the disabled on new inventions, independent living, and therapeutic advances (social, vocational, psychological, medical).

Arthritis Today: Cindy McDaniel, Managing Editor; 1314 Spring St. NW, Atlanta, GA 30309; 404-872-9559; 404-872-7100; smorrow@arthritis-erg; http://www.

arthritis.rog; circ: 20,000; bimonthly; pays $450-$1,500; 1,000-3,500 words; 45 mss/yr; byline; est: 1987; General health and lifestyle charter for arthritis sufferers focused on hobbies, recreation, and coping mechanisms with research updates, positive inspiriational recovery stories, and caretaker information.

Careers & The Disabled: James Schneider, Editor; 150 Motor Pkwy, Suite 420, Hauppauge, NY 11788-5145; 516-273-8936; 516-273-0066; circ: 12,500; 3 times/yr; pays $.10/word; 1,000-1,500 words; 15 mss/yr; byline; est: 1967; Career-guidance periodical primarily for disabled students and professionals providing job listings, job-hunting strategies, and role models for successful employment.

Deaf Life: Matthew S. Moore; 1095 Meigs Street, Rochester, NY 14620; 716-442-6371 (TTY); 716-442-6370; circ: 25,000; monthly; varies; varies; 2 mss/issue; byline; est: 1990; Tailored for and about deaf people covering entertainment, latest trends in social life and relationships, with focus on independent functioning.

Diabetes Self-Management: James Hazlett, Editor; 150 W. 22nd St., Ste. 800, New York, NY 10011-2421; 212-989-4786; 212-989-0200; circ: 285,000; monthly; pays $400-$600; 2,000-4,000 words; 10-12 mss/yr; byline; est: 1983; Health care forum for managing diabetes with focus on self-care products, latest research trends, excercise, nutrition, mental health, travel, and independence.

Mainstream: William Stothers, Editor; 2973 Beech St, San Diego, CA 92102; 619-234-3155; 619-234-3138; wstothers@aol.com; http://widow mainstream mag. com; circ: 18,200; 10 times/yr; byline; Targets active, upscale adults with disabilities including articles on employment, education, equal access, ADA legislation, personal upbeat stories, travel, and recreation.

New Mobility: Jean Dobbs, Managing Editor; 23815 Stuart Ranch Road, Malibu, CA 90265-8987; 310-317-9644; 310-317-4522; sam@miramar.com; circ: 32,000; monthly; byline; For individuals with mobility impairments, families, and rehabilitation professionals on medical and treatment options for spinal cord injury, multiple sclerosis, post-polio amputation, cerebral palsy, and muscular dystrophy.

Ethnic and Minorities

A Magazine: Joanne Chen, Features Editor; 270 Lafayette Street #400, New York, NY 10012; 212-925-2896; 212-925-4398; amag@inch.com; circ: 100,000; bimonthly; byline; Covers Asian American community with news, reviews film, finance, social issues, and psychological profiles.

AIM Magazine: Dr. Myron Apilado, Editor; 7308 S. Eberhart Ave, Chicago, IL 60620-0554; 312-874-6184; quarterly; pays $25-$35; 500-800 words; byline; est: 1975; Highlights avenues for racial harmony through arts, societal success, history/nostalgia, and toward future for high school, college, and general readers.

American Visions: Joanne Harris, Editor; 2101 S Street, Washington DC 20008; 212-496-9851; 202-462-9593; 72662.2631@compuserve.com; circ: 1986; bimonthly; pays $100-$400; 500-2,500 words; 60-70 mss/yr; byline; est: 1986; Editorial focus is on African-American art, culture, history, objectively reporting latest trends for ages 25 to 54, including books, general interest, and lifestyle.

BET Plaza: Florestine Purnell, Managing Editor; Emerge; 1900 W Place NE, Washington DC 20018; 202-608-2598; 202-608-2000; 73361.761@compuserve.com; circ: 133,507; monthly; pays $1,170-$3,000; 2,000-4,000 words; 400-600 features/yr; byline; Tabloid for educated, affluent African-Americans offering insights on government, law, society, civil rights, largely from authoritative sources.

Ebony Magazine: Lerone Bennett, Editor; 820 S. Michigan Ave., Chicago, IL 60690-2190; 312-322-9200; circ: 1 million; monthly; pays $200 min; 1,500 words max; byline; Black-oriented focused magazine exploring education and history, entertainment and arts, health, sports and social events, with book reviews.

General Consumer

The Atlantic: Cullen Murphy, Editor; 745 Boylston St., Boston, MA 02116; 617-536-9500; circ: 500,000; monthly; varies; 1,000-6,000 words; byline; For affluent readers on timely investigative reporting of news and entertainment with featured profiles of celebrities, cultural and economic trends, and some fiction and poetry.

Christian Science Monitor: Editor; 1 Norway St., Boston, MA 02115; 617-450-2000; circ: 95,000; weekly; pays $150-200; 400-900 words; byline; est: 1908; Nonsensationalistic forum for humanistic and thoroughly researched stories in fields of education, arts, environment, food, science, and technology written for upscale, advanced-degreed readership.

Friendly Exchange: Adele Malott, Editor; PO Box 2120, Warren, MI 48090-2120; 702-786-7419; circ: 5.7 million; quarterly; pays $500-$1,000; 600-1,500 words; 8 mss/yr; byline; est: 1981; Lively, colorful survey of domestic travel and leisure topics for average families from Ohio to California, covering healthy and safety, heritage and education, and facts for new products.

Grit: Michael Scheibach, Editor; 1503 SW 42nd St., Topeka, KS 66609-1265; 913-274-4300; circ: 400,000; monthly; pays $150-$500; 1,500-2,000 words; byline; est: 1882; Cornerstone magazine over a decade old for old-fashioned friendliness and down-to-earth ideas on social, family values addressing rural living, featuring home and health personal stories.

Hemispheres: Kate Greer, Editor in Chief; 1301 Carolina Street, Greensboro, NC 27401; circ: 500,000; monthly; 2,000-2,500 words; 30 features/yr; byline; est: 1992; Buys thought-provoking, informative, and entertaining pieces for professionals traveling United Airlines.

Newsweek: Maynard Parker, Editor; 251 W. 57th Street, New York, NY 10019-6999; 212-445-5068; 212-445-4000; new150a@prodigy.com; circ: 3 million; weekly; pays $1,000+; 1000 words; byline; Reporting news, commentary, opinions dealing with political and social trends, health and science discoveries, and affairs of Washington scene.

The Star: Richard Kaplan, Editor; 660 White Plains Rd., Tarrytown, NY 10591; 914-332-5043; 914-332-5000; circ: 2.8 million; weekly; pays $50-$1,500; 500-1,000 words; byline; est: 1974; Tabloid expose on family, women, and any topic affecting modern America sensationally highlighted for impulsive-buying readership.

The Sun: Sy Safransky, Editor; 107 N. Roberson St., Chapel Hill, NC 27516; 919-942-5282; circ: 27,000; weekly; pays $100-$500; 8,000 words max; byline; est: 1974; interest tabloid filled with opinion, essay, personal experience, spirituality, and latest controversy or gossip sweeping nation or in celebritihood.

Time: Jim Gaines, Managing Editor; Time-Life Bldg., Rockefeller Center, New York, NY 10020; 212-522-0323; 212-522-2955; ped@welldot.com; circ: 4 million; weekly; byline; Forum to keep readers on track with national and international news events with highlights on religion, education, law, the nation, modern living, entertainment, and changing social trends

UFO Sightings: Timothy Green Beckley, Editor; 1700 Broadway, New York, NY 10019; 212-245-1241; 212-541-7100; circ: 59,624; quarterly; byline; Covers eyewitness accounts of UFO sightings and alien abductions/encounters with personal stories, expert opinion, and updated research on unexplained phenomena.

USA Weekend: Leslie Ansley, Editor; 1000 Wilson Blvd., Arlington, VA 22229; circ: 15 million; weekly; pays $75-$2,000; 50-2,000 words; 200 mss/yr; byline; est: 1985; Newspaper magazine insert blending lively family-issue articles with timely pieces on travel, recreation, food, celebrity profile for broadly based middle America.

Health and Fitness

American Fitness: Peg Jordan, Editor; 15250 Ventura Blvd, Suite 200, Sherman Oaks, CA 91403-3297; 818-990-5468; 818-990-5468; circ: 29,000; bimonthly; byline; Fitness professionals and aerobics enthusiasts covering nutrition, exercise trends, research, and products affecting health.

American Health Magazine: Mary Witherell, Managing Editor; 28 W. 23rd St., New York, NY 10010-5204; 212-366-8760; 212-366-8900; circ: 827,643; monthly; pays $750-$3,750; 1,500-3,000 words; 60 features/yr; byline; For baby boomers intrigued with personal and physical fitness, nutrition, self-improvement.

Aspire: Mary Hopkins, Editor; 404 BNA Drive, #508, B1, Nashville, TN 37217; 615-889-0427; 615-872-8080; circ: 120,000; monthly; byline; Focuses on physical, mental, emotional, and spiritual well-being of individuals and families.

Body, Mind, Spirit Magazine: Jane Kuhn, Editor; 255 Hope Street, Providence, RI 02906; 401-272-5767; 401-351-4320; bmswriter@aol.com; circ: 150,000; 6 times/yr; pays $.20/word; 1,000 words; byline; est: 1983; Forum for personal improvement for men and women looking for practical, creative tools for body, mind, prosperity, and metaphysical direction. Informative, helpful articles with positive beat.

Cooking Light: Nathalie Dearing, Editor; Box 1748, Birmingham, AL 35201-1681; 205-877-6000; circ: 1.2 million; bimonthly; pays $250-$2,000; 400-2,000 words; 150 mss/yr; byline; est: 1987; Upbeat magazine on nutrition, healthy recipes, fitness and sports, and lifestyle nirvana through regularity of personal emotional care.

Eating Well: Marcelle Langan DiFalco, Editor; Ferry Road, Box 1001, Charlotte, Vermont 05445; 802-425-3307; 802-425-3961; ewelledit@aol.com; circ: 633,179; bimonthly; pays $1/word; 2,000 words; 12 features/yr; byline; Innovative stories from experts and personal collections interested in food, nutrition, and health.

Energy Times: Gerard McIntee, Editor; 548 Broadhollow Rd, Melville, NY 11747; 516-293-0349; 516-777-7777; circ: 575,000; bimonthly; pays $300; 1,500-2,500 words; 36 mss/yr; byline; est: 1989; Content presents articles on how to enhance life through nutrition, skin care, health maintenance, food energy sources, and products in natural market.

FIT Magazine: Lisa Goldstein, Editor; GCR Publishing, 1700 Broadway, 34th Fl, New York, NY 10019-5905; 212-245-1241; 212-541-7100; circ: 250,000; 6 times/year; pays $.50/word; 1,000-2,000 words; 10-15 mss/yr; byline; est: 1995; Reports state-of-the-art diets, exercise, nutrition and beautfy care trends and techniques, plus geared for young, active individuals oriented to improving physical self.

Health: Barbara Paulsen, Editor; 301 Howard St. #1800, San Francisco, CA 94105; 415-512-9600; 415-512-9100; reflexes@health.com; circ: 900,000; 7 times/yr; pays $1,800; 1,200 words; 25 mss/yr; byline; est: 1987; Guide for people who take charge of their own health, with regular features on money, travel, food, beauty, behavior, and fitness.

Heart & Soul: Claire McIntosh, Editor; Rodale, 733 Third Ave, 15th Floor, New York, NY 10017; 212-338-9076; 212-338-9367; circ: 200,000; bimonthly; pays $.75/word; 1,000-2,000 words; 36 mss/yr; byline; Magazine for Afro-American women discussing wellness of body, mind, and spirit and covering diet, fashion, stress management, and self-care relative to black community.

Let's Live Magazine: Beth Salmon, Editor; 320 N. Larchmont Blvd. Box 74908, Los Angeles, CA 90004; 213-469-9597; 213-469-8379; letslive@caprica.com; circ: 125,048; monthly; pays $200; 1,200-1,400 words; 2-4 mss/issue; byline; est: 1933; Information on natural dieting, including tips on preventive medicine, diet, longevity, health foods, and physical fitness. Features guides and self-help enhancers.

Listen Magazine: Anita Jacobs, Editor; 55 W. Oak Ridge Dr., Hagerstown, MD 21740; 301-790-9734; 301-791-7000; circ: 70,000; monthly; pays $.05-$.07/word; 1,200-1,500 words; 15-20 mss/yr; byline; Lifeline for recovery-spirited readers in high school, college, and professionals providing current antidrug slogans, researched articles, and inspirational alternatives for boosting self-esteem from teenage/higher points of view.

Longevity: Susan Millar Perry, Editor; 277 Park Ave, 4th Floor, New York, NY 10172-0003; 212-702-6262; 212-702-6000; longmag@aol.com; circ: 350,164; monthly; pays $100-$2,500; 150-2,000 words; byline; est: 1989; Health and lifestyle covering field of life extension with updates on health, scientific discoveries, and ways to foster wellness.

Positive Living: Elizabeth Peale Allen, Editor; PO Box 8002, Pawling, NY 12564-1409; 914-855-1462; 914-855-5000; circ: 70,000; bimonthly; byline; Extolls the power of positive thinking in inspirational articles and stories to enlighten and improve mental attitude.

Prevention: Lewis Vaughn, Managing Editor; 33 E. Minor Street, Emmaus, PA 18098-0099; 610-967-8963; 610-967-5171; markb43129@aol.com; circ: 3 million; monthly; byline; Styled for readers interested in good health through food products, meal planning, skin care, body care, and mental improvement.

Recovery Times: Ann E. Taylor, Editor; 4520 Summer Avenue, #3, Box 202, Memphis, TN 38122; 901-324-0606; 901-327-9080; circ: 119,000; monthly; byline; For individuals recovering from various addictions, focusing on healthy lifestyles, mental, emotional, and physical recuperation, and interviews with professionals.

Shape Magazine: Nancy Gottesman, Features Editor; 21100 Erwin St., Woodland Hills, CA 91367-3712; 818-704-5734; 818-595-0492; circ: 804,764; monthly; 500-2,000 words; byline; est: 1981; Essential outlet for contemporary, active women who emphasize fitness, healthy lifestyle, and want latest trends in self-help, exercise, travel, and romance.

Sober Times: Gerald D. Miller, Editor; 6306 E. Green Lake Way, North, Seattle, WA 98103; 206-523-8085; circ: 75,000; bimonthly; pays $50+; 900-2,000 words; 90 mss/yr; byline; est: 1987; Tabloid on alcohol and substance abuse recovery with personal stories and expert advice on championing sobriety for healthy lifestyles.

Vibrant Life: Larry Becker, Editor; 55 W. Oak Ridge Dr., Hagerstown, MD 21740-7301; 301-790-9734; 301-791-7000; circ: 50,000; bimonthly; pays $125-$250; 750-1,800 words; 20-25 mss/yr; byline; est: 1845; Promotes quality of life through focus on proper nutrition, exercise, mental and emotional health, and positive family relationships with respect to faith in God. Uses natural principles for good health.

Vim & Vigor: Fred Petrovsky, Editor; 8805 N. 23rd Ave, Suite 400, Phoenix, AZ 85021-4171; 602-395-5853; 602-395-5850; circ: 900,000; quarterly; pays $500;

2,000 words; 4 mss/yr; byline; est: 1985; Health-conscious individual covering diagnosis and treatment of medical conditions from doctor's and patient's standpoint on diet, fitness, and emotional and physical health.

Weight Watchers Magazine: Nancy Gagliardi, Editor; 360 Lexington Ave, 11th Floor, New York, NY 10017-6547; 212-687-4398; 212-370-0644; circ: 1 million; monthly; pays $700; 1,500 words; 12 mss/issue; byline; est: 1968; Explores women's healthy from overall weight loss perspective, focused on health, fitness, and self-improvement.

The Yoga Journal: Rick Fields, Editor; 2054 University Ave., Suite 601, Berkeley, CA 94704-1082; 510-644-3101; 510-841-9200; circ: 86,000; bimonthly; pays $1,000-$1,200; features; 3,500-5,000 words; 5-6 mss/issue; byline; est: 1975; Vehicle to communicate principles of yoga including peace, integrity, clarity, and compassion. Focus on mind-body conection and personal and spiritual development, oriented to holistic healing and transpersonal psychology.

Your Health: Susan Gregg, Editor; 5401 NW Broken Sound Blvd, Boca Raton, FL 33487; 407-997-9210; 407-997-7733; yhealth@aol.com; circ: 50,000; biweekly; pays $25-$150; 300-2,000 words; 75-100 mss/yr; byline; est: 1962; Geared for natural health-improving public with self-help articles on current medical research and reports related to personal health care written by specialists.

Juvenile

Boy's Life: J.D. Owen, Managing Editor; PO Box 152079, Irving, TX 75015-2079; circ: 1.3 million; monthly; pays $400-$1,500; 500-1,500 words; 85 features/yr; byline; est: 1911; Boys adventure and interest articles for readers ages 8 to 18, focusing on sports, science, aviation, high-tech, and personal health made easy.

Boys' Quest: Marilyn Edwards, Editor; 103 North Main, Bluffton, OH 45817; 419-358-5027; 419-358-4610; circ: 4,000; bimonthly; pays $.05/word; 500-700 words; 60-80 mss/yr; byline; est: 1995; Thematic periodical tracking trends for young contemporary boys' lives from recreation to self-exploring to games and puzzles.

Healthy Kids Magazine: Laura Broadwell, Editor; 249 W. 17th Street, New York, NY 10011; 212-463-6410; 212-463-6578; circ: 1.5 million; bimonthly; pays $750-$1,000; 1,500-2,500 words; 5 features/issue; byline; est: 1989; Parenting magazine devoted to the health issues of children birth through age 10.

Highlights for Children: Beth Troop, Manuscript Coordinator; 803 Church St., Honesdale, PA 18431-1824; 717-253-0179; 717-253-1080; circ: 2.5 million; monthly; varies; 800 words; byline; est: 1946; Printed for children ages 2 to 12 with stories, nonfiction articles on science, games, and fun activities. Issues cover healthy behavior, tips for development, and use of analytical and vocabulary skills.

Hopscotch: Marilyn Edwards, Editor; 103 N. Main Street, Bluffton, OH 45817; 419-358-5027; 419-358-4610; circ: 10,000; bimonthly; pays $.05/word; 500-700 words; 60-80 mss/yr; byline; est: 1989; Edited for preteen females to stimulate interest in scientific and technologic vocations, with emphasis on literacy, comprehension skills, positive principles for role models, and teaching tools for healthy growth.

Humpty Dumpty's Magazine: Sandra J. Grieshop, Editor; PO Box 567, Indianapolis, IN 46206-0567; 317-684-8094; 317-636-8881; circ: 264,742; 8 times/yr; pays $.22/word; 500 words; 60 mss/yr; byline; est: 1989; Created for 4- to 6-year-olds, featuring imaginative stories and articles on health, nutrition, safety, positive peer relations.

Jack and Jill: Daniel Lee, Editor; 1100 Waterway Blvd., Indianapolis, IN 46202-2156; 317-637-0126; 317-636-8881; circ: 334,212; 8 times/yr; pays $.15/word; 500-800 words; 10-15 mss/yr; byline; Targeted for 7 to 10 age group with articles, games, humor, all for raising appetite for enriching fun and learning.

You!: Paul Lauer, Editor; 31194 La Baya, #200, Westlake Village, CA 91362; 818-991-2024; 818-991-1813; youmag@earthlink.com; circ: 35,000; monthly; $.07/word; 1,000 words; 10 mss/yr; byline; est: 1987; Channeled for Catholic and Christian teenagers and young adults with goal of fusing gap between popular culture and religion through self-enhancing language and ways of relating to world. Format features entertainment and self-help.

Men and Sexuality

Bachelorette Book: Paul Gallotta, Senior Editor; 8222 Wiles Road, Suite 111, Coral Springs, FL 33067; 305-341-8982; 305-341-8801; circ: 25,000; quarterly; byline; Trendy, contemporary lifestyle magazine featuring single gentlemen of the 1990s in relationships, romance, and for eligibility for women.

Details: Joe Levy, Features Editor; Details; 632 Broadway, New York, NY 10012; 212-228-0674; 212-598-3710; detailsmag@aol.com; circ: 476,145; monthly; pays $.075-$1.00/word; 3,000-5,000 words; 60 features/yr; byline; Encourages creative look at style, sex, cultural trends, news, sports, and romance for men ages 18 to 34.

Ebony Man: Willie Wofford Jr., Managing Editor; 820 S. Michigan Avenue, Chicago, IL 60605-2103; 312-322-0178; 312-322-9200; circ: 285,755; monthly; byline; Guide for fashion, grooming, health, and fitness of Black Men. Focus on career, relationships, nutrition, sports, and travel.

Esquire: Michael Solomon, Features Editor; 250 W. 55th St., 7th Floor, New York, NY 10019; 212-977-3158; 212-649-4253; esquire@hearst.com; circ: 739,828; monthly; pays $1/word; 6,000-8,000 words; 30 features/yr; byline; est: 1933; College educated, sophisticated men's reader on social, sexual, and career pointers.

Gallery Magazine: Rich Friedman, Editor; 401 Park Ave. S, New York, NY 10016-8802; 212-725-7215; 212-779-8900; circ: 400,000; monthly; pays $300-

$1,500; 1,000-3,000 words; 4-5 mss/issue; byline; est: 1972; Entertainment magazine for men emphasizing the pleasures, politics, and events shaping current lifestyles and romances, with departments on new product reviews and arts, sports.

Genesis: Steve Glassman, Editor; 110 E. 59th St., Suite 3100, New York, NY 10022; 212-644-9212; 212-644-8800; circ: 400,000; 13 times/yr; pays $100-$500; 1,500-2,000 words; 65 mss/yr; byline; est: 1973; Geared to male readers, stressing heterosexual relationships, news, entertainment, and personal contentment.

Gentlemen's Quarterly: Lisa Henricksson, Features Editor; 350 Madison Avenue, New York, NY 10017-3704; 212-880-8757; 212-880-8800; gqmag@aol.com; circ: 658,346; monthly; varies; 1,500-4,000 words; 4-6 mss/issue; byline; Traditional men's articles on fashion, dating, personality profiles, and politics.

Hustler: Allan MacDonell, Editor; 9171 Wilshire Blvd., Ste. 900, Los Angeles, CA 90211; 213-651-1289; 213-651-5400; circ: 1 million; monthly; pays $1,000; 3,500-4,000 words; 30 mss/yr; byline; est: 1974; Serves male audience featuring celebrities and stories on contemporary society, politics, humor, and entertainment, with photo-essays.

Inside Edge: Matt Leinwohl, Editor; 258 Harvard Street, #329, Brookline, MA 02146; 617-739-7071; 617-739-5067; circ: 125,000; 10 times/yr; byline; Targets young men ages 18 to 24 focusing on sports, socializing, fitness, and adventure, and contains practical advice on spending quality, romantic time.

Men's Fitness: Chris Bennett, Administrative Assistant; 21100 Erwin Street, Woodland Hills, CA 91367-3712; 818-704-5734; 818-884-6800; circ: 306,485; monthly; pays $500-$1,000; 1,000-1,800 words; byline; est: 1987; For active men who view healthy living as essential to careers, family relationships, covering stress and time management, fitness, nutrition, and self-improvement.

Men's Health: Stephen Perrine, Articles Editor; 33 E. Minor Street, Emmaus, PA 18098-4113; 610-967-7725; 610-967-5171; menshlth@msn.com; circ: 1 million; 10 times/yr; byline; Assist men who are attuned to health, careers, family, and sexual relationships, fitness, nutrition, and leisure activities.

Men's Perspective: Trevor Miller, Editor; 5670 Wilshire Blvd, #1240, Los Angeles, CA 90036; 213-965-0915; 213-965-7800; circ: 150,000; monthly; byline; Covers trends for contemporary single men searching for healthy relationships and lifestyle variety.

Men's Style: C. Bard Cole, Managing Edtior; 55 Fifth Avenue, New York, NY 10003; 212-924-3194; 212-924-3000; mensmag@aol.com; bimonthly; varies; 4-6 mss/issue; byline; est: 1995; Loyal to lifestyle, romance, and professional lifestyle of gay men.

New Man: Brian Peterson, Editor; 600 Rinehart Road, Lake Mary, FL 32746; 407-333-7133; 407-333-0600; circ: 225,000; bimonthly; byline; Devoted to growing number of men who made lifetime commitment to holiness, reconciliation, and discipleship. Covers aspects of lifestyle–spiritual, physical, emotional, and social.

Penthouse: Peter Bloch, Editor; 277 Park Ave, 4th Floor, New York, NY 10172-0003; 212-702-6279; 212-702-6000; pentedit@aol.com; circ: 1 million; monthly; pays $1,000+; 1,000+; 3 mss/issue; byline; est: 1969; Sophisticated male focus on outspoken contemporary issues and in-depth coverage of personalities, sociological studies, humor, travel, romance, and grooming for men. Focus on nonfiction.

Playboy: John Rezek, Features Editor; 680 N. Lake Shore Drive, 16th Floor, Chicago, IL 60611-3088; 312-951-2939; 312-751-8000; edit@playboy.com; circ: 3 million; monthly; byline; High-profile men's magazine informative on music, movies, interviews on relationships, self-improvement, and celebrity profiles.

Players: Lecil Willis, Editor; 8060 Melrose Avenue, Los Angeles, CA 90046-7017; 213-655-9452; 213-653-8060; circ: 175,000; monthly; byline; Upbeat news and contemporary stories for modern Black male focused on lifestyle, careers, and relationships with women.

Swank: Palu Gambino, Editor; 210 Route 4, East #401, Paramus, NJ 07652; 201-843-8636; 201-843-4004; circ: 325,000; 13 times/yr; pays $350-$500; 34 mss/yr; byline; est: 1954; Content emphasizes investigative reporting on humor, sex, with regular departments on food, wine, equipment, and fashion essays of women.

Military

Off Duty Magazine: Gary Burch, Editor; 3303 Harbor Blvd, Suite 10, Costa Mesa, CA 92626-1500; 714-549-4222; 714-549-7172; circ: 450,000; bimonthly; pays $160-$420; 800-1,200 words; 30-40 mss/yr; byline; est: 1970; Leisure time magazine for personnel throughout the world, focused on on-base shopping, food, and dining, lifetyle issues concerning individuals and family.

Reunions Magazine: Edith Wagner, Editor; PO Box 11727, Milwaukee, WI 53211-0727; 414-263-4567; 414-263-6331; reunions@execpc.com; circ: 18,000; quarterly; pays $25; 16-20 mss/yr; byline; est: 1990; Only resource entirely devoted to announcing and guiding persons organizing family and reunions.

Self-Help

Changes: Jeffrey Laign, Managing Editor; 3201 SW 15th Street, Deerfield Beach, FL 33442-8190; 305-360-0034; 800-851-9100; bimonthly; 1,000 words; 5-6 mss/issue; byline; For people radically changing their lives and cultivating inner well-being and physical health through intimate relationships, spiritual insights, capable to confront family issues related to alcohol, drug, and sexual abuse.

Professional Counselor: Richard Fields, PhD, Editor; 3201 Southwest 15th Street, Deerfield Beach, FL 33442-8190; 305-360-0034; 800-851-9100; bimonthly; 5 features/issue; byline; Mainstream magazine featuring cutting edge articles by clinicians on recovery methods and process of alcohol and drug abuse rehabilitation.

Psychology Today: Sunny Edmonds, Managing Editor; 49 E. 21st Street, 11th Floor, New York, NY 10010; 212-260-7445; 212-260-7210; psychtoday@aol.com; circ: 350,000; bimonthly; byline; Emphasizes human behavior relating to current trends affecting physical health, personal relationships, nutrition, and exercise, and offering new psychological theories.

10 Percent: Steve Petrow, Editor; 54 Mint Street, #200, San Francisco, CA 94103-1819; 415-227-0463; 415-905-8590; editor10@eworld.com; relationship; circ: 22,000; bimonthly; byline; For lesbian, gay, and bisexual community in and around University of Califorinia at Los Angeles, offering thoughts on social, political, and personality profiles.

Relationships

Advocate: Bruce Wright, Features Editor; PO Box 4371, Los Angeles, CA 90078-4371; 213-467-6805; 213-871-1225; newsroom@advocate.com; circ: 75,000; biweekly; byline; National news tabloid edited for gay men and lesbians including opinions, investigative reporting, humor, reviews, political, and legal commentary and advice on medical, social, and sexual aspects of lifestyle.

Atlantic Singles: Shannon McClintock, Editor; 180 Allen Rd., Suite 304N, Atlanta, GA 30328; 404-256-9719; 404-256-9411; circ: 15,000; bimonthly; pays $50-$150; 600-1,200 words; 5 mss/yr; byline; est: 1977; Hotline for single, widowed, divorced adults in professional, stable careers oriented to longlasting relationships, featuring fashion, investment, marriage, sexuality.

Bliss: Swami Virato, Editor; Box 17397, Asheville, NC 28806; circ: 10,000; quarterly; pays $50-$150; byline; est: 1993; Publishes personal profiles and expert opinion on sex and spirituality (not pornography) with inspirational slant on metaphysics.

First Hand: Bob Harris, Editor; 310 Cedar Lane, Teaneck, NJ 07666; 201-836-5055; 201-836-9177; circ: 70,000; monthly; pays $35-$70; 1,000 words; byline; est: 1980; Outlet for homosexual exploration of erotica covering sensuality related to psychology, taboos (bestiality, rape, etc.), and gay lifestyle.

Guys: William Spencer, Editor; BOX 1314, Teaneck, NJ 07666-3441; 201-836-5055; 201-836-9177; circ: 60,000; monthly; pays $75-$100; 1,250-1,500; 36 mss/yr; byline; est: 1988; Positive, romantic articles for gay men into erotica and seeking latest in arts and entertainment, and upbeat emphasis on lifestyle.

Single Styles: Robert Yehling, Editor; PO Box 1257, Largo, FL 34649; 813-593-0539; 813-595-5008; circ: 125,000; monthly; byline; Targeted to single adults with advice on parenting, success, recreational ideas, technology, and entertainment. Large focus on art of single living.

Swing Magazine: Rob Speyer, Senior Editor; 342 Madison Avenue, #1402, New York, NY 10017; 212-490-8073; 212-490-0525; circ: 100,000; 10 times/yr; byline; Designed for today's 18 to 25 upperly mobile men and women on topics as music, fashion, social problems, and success.

Religion

Discipleship: Jonathan Graf, Managing Editor; Box 35004, Colorado Springs, CO 80935; 719-598-7128; 719-548-9222; smaycini@navigato.mhs.compuserve. com; circ: 100,000; bimonthly; pays $.20/word; 1,500-2,000 words; 40 features/yr; byline; est: 1981; Articles enhancing Christian development, practical help in family interpretation and daily life; evangelism, prayer, and forming intimacy with God.

The Family: Sr. Theresa Frances, Editor; 50 St. Paul's Ave., Boston, MA 02130; 617-522-8911; monthly; pays $50-$125; 500-1,500 words; 20 mss/yr; byline; est: 1952; Stresses Catholic family values in pertinent issues incorporating faith into love, society, and childcare, written with spiritual basis.

Family Scrapbook: Ginger Kauffman, Editor; 9943 Wesley Road, Houghton, NY 14744; 716-567-2608; circ: 12,700; bimonthly; byline; Focuses on inspirational subjects affecting Christian families, with useful ideas for health and money.

Journal of Christian Camping: Dean Ridings, Editor; PO Box 62189, Colorado Springs, CO 80962-2189; 719-260-6398; 719-260-9400, ext. 15; cciusa@usa.pipeline.com; circ: 7,000; bimonthly; pays $.06/word; 1,000-1,250 words; byline; Flagship publication of CCI/USA . It provides helpful articles, insightful perspectives, and product, service, and resource information for outdoor ministries and Christian hospitality.

Our Sunday Visitor Magazine: David Scott, Editor; 200 Noll Plaza, Huntington IN 46750-4304; 219-356-8472; 219-356-8400; 76440,3571@compuserve.com; relig; circ: 130,000; monthly; pays $100+; 1,000-1,200 words; 25 mss/yr; byline; Spotlights news and activities for church members and parishoners on health, psychology, and events affecting the Catholic Church.

Vibrant Life: Larry Becker, Editor; 55 W. Oak Ridge Drive, Hagerstown, MD 21740; bimonthly; pays $75-$250; 500-1,500 words; 50-60 features/yr; byline; Variety of family and health topics with Christian perspective.

Virtue: Jeanette Thomason, Editor; 4050 Lee Vance View, Colorado Springs, CO 80918; 719-535-0172; 719-531-7776; relig; circ: 115,000; bimonthly; pays $.15-$.25/word; 600-1,800 words; 60 mss/yr; byline; est: 1978; Features articles on marriage, family, self-esteem, work, and home in lives of Christian women.

Retirement

Active Times Magazine: Chris Kelly, Editor; 417 Main St., Carbondale, CO 81623; circ: 7 million; quarterly; pays $75-$1,000; 500-2,000 words; 50 mss/yr; byline; est: 1992; Highlights active adults over 50 in recreationally high-profile activity, covering travel, sports and fitness, nostalgia, history.

A Better Tomorrow: Vicki Huffman, Editor; 404 BNA Dr., Ste. 508, Bldg 200, Nashville,TN 37217; 615-872-8080; circ: 20,000; bimonthly; pays $60-$400; 800-3,000 words; 10-15 mss/yr; byline; est: 1992; Inspires encouraging pieces for baby boomers now raising children and retrospetive look at changing society, with story anecdotes on grandchildren all oriented from Christian perspective.

Fifty Plus: Linda Scovill, Editor; 314 Bush Drive, Myrtle Beach, SC 29577; 803-235-3602; monthly; byline; For adults over 50 geared toward more active and affluent individuals on legislation, travel, and self-sustaining health and mind tips.

Florida Style: Kerry Smith, Editor; Box 161848, Altamonte Springs, FL 32714-1848; 407-774-9069; 407-774-8668; circ: 50,000; monthly; pays $.10/word; 800-1,500 words; 30 mss/yr; byline; est: 1946; Addresses housing, community living, planning, recreation, lifestyle enhancement for Florida men.

Golden Times: Carmen Viglucci, Editor; 80 Rockwood Place; Rochester, NY 14610; 716-256-2765; 716-242-9930; circ: 20,000; semi-monthly; byline; Active, affluent older adults informed of a variety of issues from book reviews, finance, travel, recreation, health, with focus on self-improvement and legislation.

Grandparenting and Other Great Adventures: Vicki Huffman, Editor; 404 BNA Drive, #600, Bldg. 200, Nashville, TN 37217; 615-889-0437; 615-872-8080; circ: 50,000; bimonthly; byline; Christian perspective on health, nutrition, fitness, finances, and spiritual growth for grandparents looking forward to the future.

Mature Living: Al Shackleford, Editor; 127 9th Avenue North, Nashville, TN 37234-0140; 615-251-5008; 615-251-2191; monthly; byline; Readers ages 50+ adopting a Christian lifestyle receive positive, inspirational stories and messages on living powerful golden years.

Mature Outlook: Peggy Person, Editor; 1912 Grand Ave., Des Moines, IA 50309-3379; 515-284-2007; circ: 931,813; bimonthly; pays $100-$750; 150-1,000 words; 50-60 mss/yr; byline; Created for vibrant over 50 featuring contemporary coverage on food, travel, health, fitness, money, and life betterment tips.

Mature Years: Marvin Cropsey, Editor; 201 Eigth Ave. S., Nashville, TN 37202-0801; 615-749-6512; circ: 70,000; quarterly; pays $45-$125; 900-2,500 words; 75-80 mss/yr; byline; est: 1954; Forum for older adults nearing retirement years wanting resources for Christian faith related to issues of aging.

Modern Maturity: John Wood, Features Editor; AARP; 601 E. Street NW, Washington, DC 20049; (202) 434-6880; circ: 33 million; bimonthly; pays up to $3,000; 2,000 words; byline; Official voice of AARP with broad coverage for age

50+ readers of financial planning, health, and psychology, careers, and socialpolitical issues.

Senior Highlights: Lee McCamon, Editor; 26081 Merit Circle, Suite 101, Laguna Hills CA 92653-7015; 714-367-1006; 714-367-0776; circ: 444,000; monthly; pays $25; 300-800 words; 60 mss/yr; byline; est: 1983; For and about active adults over 50 focused on vacation, keeping fit, entertainment, money, and retirement lifestyles with upbeat attitude.

Senior Magazine: Gary D. Suggs, Editor; 3565 S. Higuera Street, San Luis Obispo, CA 93401-7394; 805-544-4450; 805-544-8711; circ: 247,000; monthly; pays $1.50/word; 300-900 words; 30-75 mss/yr; byline; est: 1981; Highlights financial affairs, legal, health, housing, leisure-time activities for over 50 regional population.

Sports

Adventure Cyclist: Dan D'Ambrosio, Editor; Adventure Cyclist; 150 East Pine Street, Missoula, MT 59802; 406-721-8754; 406-721-1776; acabike@aol.com; circ: 40,000; 9 times/yr; pays $250; 1,200-3,500 words; 3 features/issue; byline; est: 1976; Magazine devoted to international bicycle travel tailored to Adventure Cycling Association membership showing destinations, attitude, inspirational stories, new product resources and reviews.

Field & Stream: Cathleen Meyers, Editor; 2 Park Ave, New York, NY 10016-5695; 212-725-3836; 212-779-5000; circ: 2 million; monthly; pays $800+; 1,500-2,000 words; byline; est: 1895; For outdoor enthusiasts especially hunters and fisherman, with how-to articles on humor, mood pieces, new products, and safety.

Hockey Player Magazine: Alex Carswell, Editor; PO Box 312, Okemos, MI 48864; 517-347-0686; 517347-1172; hockeymag@aol.com; circ: 35,000; monthly; pays $50-$75; 1750-2,250 words; 5 mss/issue; byline; est: 1991; Tailored for youth and adults in recreational hockey featuring how-to articles on game improvement and positive mental attitude.

Metro Magazine: Miles Jaffe, Editor; 27 W. 24th Street, #10B, New York, NY 10010; 212-627-7446; 212-627-7040; metrosport@aol.com; circ: 250,000; 10 times/yr; pays $.15/word; 800-1,500 words; 8 features/month; byline; est: 1990; Focuses on skating, tennis, skiing, and running with features on health, fitness, sport therapies, vacation resorts, adventure travel, and events affecting currents of these. Frequently read while person on treadmill or stairmaster.

Surfer Magazine: Sam George, Managing Editor; PO Box 1028, Dana Point, CA 92629; 714-496-7849; 714-496-5922; surferedit@aol.com; circ: 105,000; monthly; pays $.20 to $.30/word; 400 to 3,000 words; 3 mss/issue; byline; est: 1960; For dedicated surfers to identify ecstatic pleasures and skillful trade tips of the sport.

Travel

Camping Today: DeWayne Johnston, Editor; 126 Hermitage Rd., Butler, PA 16001-8509; 412-283-6401; circ: 25,000; monthly; pays $50-$150; 750-2,000 words; 10-15 mss/yr; byline; est: 1983; Family travel experiences.

Carlson Voyageur: Melinda Stovall, Editor; 1301 Carolina St., Greensboro, NC 27401; circ: 150,000; quarterly; pays $300-$800; 600 words; 12 mss/yr; byline; Guest-room entertainment and travel.

Crown & Anchor: Lynn Ulivieri, Managing Editor; Crown & Anchor; 777 Arthur Godfrey Rd., Suite 300; Miami Beach, FL 33140; 305-674-9396; 305-673-0400; circ: 792,184; annual; pays $150-$1,000; 800-2,000 words; 12 features/yr; byline; est: 1992; News and for cruise line customers.

Cruise Travel Magazine: Charles Doherty, Managing Edtior; 990 Grove St, Evanston, IL 60201-4370; 708-491-0867; 708-491-6440; circ: 200,000; bimonthly; pays $100-$400; 500-1,500 words; 72 mss/yr; byline; est: 1979; Customer-oriented articles for cruise ship.

Family Motor Coaching: Pamela Wisby Kay, Editor; 8291 Clough Pike, Cincinnati, OH 45244-2796; 513-474-2332; 513-474-3622; circ: 99,000; monthly; pays $100-$500; 1,000-2,000 words; 15-20 mss/issue; byline; est: 1963; Motorhome travel topics and new products.

Journal of Christian Camping: Dean Ridings, Editor; PO Box 62189, Colorado Springs, CO 80962; 719-260-6398; 719-260-9400; cciusa@aol.com; circ: 6,500; bimonthly; pays $.06/word; 600-1,200 words; 20-30 mss/yr; byline; est: 1963; Inspirational, motivational, and stories of camping.

Mature Traveler: Gene Malott, Editor; PO Box 50400, Reno, NV 89513-0400; 702-786-7419; maturetrav@aol.com; circ: 2,500; monthly; pays $50-$100; 600-1,200 words; byline; est: 1984; Pieces on seniors travelling and destinations.

RV Times Magazine: Tom Rigney, Editor; 1100 Welbourne Dr., Suite 204, Richmond, VA 23229; 804-741-9659; 804-741-5376; circ: 35,000; monthly; 500-2,000 words; 80 mss/yr; byline; est: 1973; How-to and travel information for camping.

Travel & Leisure: Barbara Peck, Executive Editor; 1120 Avenue of the Americas, New York, NY 10036; 212-382-5877; 212-382-5600; tlquery@amexpub.com; circ: 960,000; monthly; pays $1,000-$4,000; 1,500-4,000 words; 8-10 mss/issue; byline; est: 1971; Magazine for sophisticated travel readers emphasizing destinations, upscale vacationing, and perspectives on enjoyment. For experienced writers only.

USAir Magazine: Catherin Sabino, Editor; 14th Floor, 122 E. 42nd Street, New York, NY 10168; monthly; pays $1,500-$2,000; 1,000-1,500 words; 75 features/yr; byline; Topic pieces sought on lifestyle, personality, travel for travelers of USAir.

Women's Magazines

Allure: Tom Prince, Editor; 360 Madison Ave., New York, NY 10017; 212-370-1949; 212-880-2341; alluremag@aol.com; circ: 705,666; monthly; 1,000-5,000 words; byline; Stories on romance, partnerships, life-building experiences in pre-family years.

Ambience: Deborah Fleischman, Editor; PO Box 12134, Berkeley, CA 94712; quarterly; 1,000-5,000 words; 30 mss/yr; byline; est: 1995; Focus on aged 20 and over sensuality.

American Woman: Illona Price, Features Senior Editor; 1700 Broadway, 34th Floor, New York, NY 10019-5905; 212-245-1241; 212-541-7100; circ: 149,916; monthly; pays $200-$700; 700-1,500 words; 40 mss/yr; byline; est: 1990; True-life stories/inspiration of women overcoming obstacles.

Better Homes & Garden: Larmont Olson, Managing Editor; Meredith Corporation, 1716 Locust Street, Des Moines, IA 50309-3023; 515-284-3000; circ: 2 million; monthly; byline; Tabloid profiling family lifestyles, interior and exterior home designs, decorating, and romance.

Complete Woman: Bonnie Krueger, Editor; 875 N. Michigan Ave., Chicago, IL 60611-1901; 312-266-8680; circ: 150,000; monthly; pays $80-$400; 800-2,000 words; 60-100 mss/yr; byline; est: 1980; Self-help articles for uppwardly mobile women.

Cosmopolitan: Irene Copeland, Features Editor; 224 W. 57th St, New York, NY 10019-3299; 212-956-3268; 212-649-2000; circ: 2 million; monthly; pays $800-$3,000; 2,000-3,000 words; 350 mss/yr; byline; Stories on working women aged 18 to 35 years old.

Country Woman: Kathy Pohl, Managing Editor; 5400 S. 60th Street, Greendale, WI; 414-423-3840; 414-423-0100; circ: 1 million; bimonthly; pays $75-$125; 1,000 max words; 5-24 mss/yr; byline; est: 1970; Targets women living in rural areas of United States with topics on lifestyle, gardening, decorating, cooking, historical anecdotes, and traditional, how-to country values.

Daughters of Sarah: Elizabeth Anderson, Editor; 2121 Sheridan Road, Evanston, IL 60201; 708-866-3882; circ: 5,000; quarterly; pays $15/printed page; 500-2,100 words; byline; est: 1974; Bible-based personal and feminist experiences of women.

Essence: Valerie Wilson Wesley, Editor; 1500 Broadway, New York, NY 10036-4071; 212-921-5173; 212-642-0600; circ: 1 million; monthly; pays $500 minimum; 200 mss/yr; byline; est: 1970; Black women experiences, social style and contemporary international issues explored.

Esteem Magazine: Carla Welborn, Editor; PO Box 9066, Cincinnati, OH 45209; 513-366-4412; 513-351-1790; circ: 75,000; quarterly; byline; Highlights young African-American women from ages of 12 to 24 aiming to enlighten, entertain, and educate with stories on self-reliance, self-respect, beauty, fashion, independence, and career development.

Extra Woman: Michele Durant, Editor; PO Box 57194, Sherman Oaks, CA 91413; 818-909-0758; 818-997-8404; circ: 35,000; bimonthly; byline; Created for full-figured women as forum of expression on well-being, fashion, health, medical, and psychological news and fiction.

Glamour: Ruth Whitney, Editor; 350 Madison Ave., New York, NY 10017; 212-880-6922; 212-880-8800; glamourmag@aol.com; circ: 2.3 million; monthly; pays $1,000 +; 2,500-3,000 words; 10-12 mss/yr; byline; est: 1939; Strongly interested in male-female relationships.

Hues: Susan Gilman, Editor; PO Box 7778, Ann Arbor, MI 48107-8226; 313-747-7462; 313-994-3930; leora@umich.edu; circ: 120,000; semi-annually; byline; Dedicated to enhancing self-esteem for women of all cultures, shapes, and experiences, with features on hip, hardcore, and happening women, reviews, personal profiles, and politics.

Ladies' Home Journal: Pamela O'Brien, Features Edtior; 100 Park Avenue, New York, NY 10017-5599; 212-351-3650; 212-953-7070; circ: 5 million; monthly; 1,500-3,000 words; 12 mss/yr; byline; Contemporary articles on today's women ages 30 to 45 on decorating, entertainment, fitness, nutrition, family and marriage, lifestyle trends.

Mademoiselle: Faye Haun, Managing Editor; 350 Madison Avenue, New York, NY 10017; 212-880-8289; 212-880-8800; milemag@aol.com; circ: 1.2 million; monthly; 1,000 words; byline; Addressing savvy, intelligent, uppwardly mobile and career women on social and fashion trends.

Marie Claire: Bonnie Fuller, Editor; 250 W. 55th St., New York, NY 10019; 212-541-4295 (fax); marieclaire@hearst.com; circ: 500,000; monthly; pays $1-$1.50/word; 500-3,000 words, byline; International coverage of female culture on topics of relationship, sex, self-help, career and finances, all through women's perspective.

McCall's: Catherine Cavender, Executive Editor; 110 Fifth Avenue, New York, NY 10011; 212-463-1403; 212-463-1462; circ: 5 million; monthly; pays $1.00/word; 1,200-1,500 words; 144 features/yr; byline; Oriented to women readers on fashion, parenting, food and diet, and celebrity personalities.

MS Magazine: Gloria Jacobs, Features Editor; 230 Park Avenue, 7th Floor, New York, NY 10168; 212-551-9384; 212-551-9595; ms@echonyc.com; circ: 200,000; bimonthly; pays $1,800-$4,000; 2,500-4,000; byline; Needs strong feminist reportage, profiles, investigative stories, and topics on self and health for progressive women.

New Woman: Emma Segal, Features Editor; 215 Lexington Avenue, 3rd floor, New York, NY 10016-6075; 212-251-1590; 212-251-1500; circ: 1 million; monthly; pays $1.00/word; 1,000+ words; 6-10 mss/issue; byline; est: 1970; Helps today's career-minded women stay abreast of social trends and build strengths in personal and professional relationships, coping with stress, and personal finance, integrating values of sixties and seventies.

Redbook: Harriet Lyons, Features Senior Editor; 224 West 57th Street, New York, NY 10019-3299; 212-581-8114; 212-649-3450; circ: 3.2 million; monthly; varies; 1,500-3,000; 10 features/yr; byline; est: 1903; Focused on timely topics for ages 25 to 44 on sex, marriage, money, celebrities, and social issues.

ROCKRGRL: Carla DeSantis, Editor in Chief; 7 West 41st Avenue, Suite 113, San Mateo, CA 94403; 415-573-7625; rockrgrl@aol.com; circ: 5,000; bimonthly; 900 words; byline; est: 1995; For and about women in the music industry, primarily rock. Mission is to educate, inspire, and promote networking in an industry that is often quite hostile toward women. Writers need to pitch ideas and send prior work for consideration.

Victoria: Nancy Lindemeyer, Editor; 224 West 57th Street, 4th Floor, New York, NY 10019-3203; 212-757-6109; 212-649-3720; circ: 907,034; monthly; byline; Pages of traditional, old-fashioned Victorian era topics and fashions for contemporary lifestyle.

Vogue: Susan Morrison, Features Director; 350 Madison Avenue, New York, NY 10017-3799; 212-880-8169; 212-880-8800; voguemail@aol.com; circ: 1 million; monthly; pays $1-$2 per word; 2,500 words; 36 features/yr; byline; Fresh look at contemporary woman's role in culture, hollywood, lifestyles, and gripping personal stories.

Wahine Magazine: Elizabeth A. Glazner, Editor; 5520 E. 2nd Street, Suite K, Long Beach, CA 90803; 310-434-9444; 310-434-9444; wahinemag@aol.com; circ: 25,000; quarterly; pays $50-$150; 500-1,500 words; 2 health features/yr; byline; est: 1994; Periodical covers all aspects of a healthy beach lifestyle including fitness, nutrition, and other special columns related to body and soul.

Woman's Day: Rebecca Greer, Senior Articles Editor; 1633 Broadway, New York, NY 10019; 212-767-5785; 212-767-6418; womansday@aol.com; circ: 6 million; 17 issues/yr; pays $1,500-$5,000; 500-2,500 words; 100-125 features/yr; byline; Profiles woman age 20 to 60 in crafts, food and nutrition, psychology, beauty and fashion, home design, fitness, and light romance. Personal narratives with professional slant a plus.

Woman's Own: Estelle Sobel, Editor; 1115 Broadway, New York, NY 10010; 212-627-4678; 212-807-7100; womansown@aol.com; circ: 250,000; monthly; 1,000-2,000 words; byline; Reports upbeat and current trends in relationships, sexuality, career, fashions.

Women & Fitness: Mary Duffy, Editor in Chief; 2025 Pearl Street, Boulder, CO 80304; 8 issues/yr; 1,000-2,000 words; 35 features/yr; byline; Highlights current vogues in nutrition, motivation, and health for active-minded women.

Young and Modern: Sally Lee, Editor; 685 Third Avenue, 28th Floor, New York, NY 10017-4024; 212-286-0935; 212-878-8700; circ: 2 million; 10 issues/year;

pays $.75-$1.00/word; 1,500-2,000; 50 features/yr; byline; Responds to 14 to 22 year old single-living and dating women with topics on celebrities, beauty and fitness, guy watching, self-improvement.

SOFTWARE COMPANIES

The following entries are a representative sample of software companies in business and general areas. Each entry follows a sequence of information based on the replies from each company or culled from a variety of sources. Entirely completed entries include these items:

Name of software company: address, state, zip code; president/owner; examples of software; function of software and needs of company.

The format changes slightly for general retail software companies and is described under that category.

Human Resources Software Companies

Affirmative Action/EEOC Records

Berkshire Associates Incorporated: 8930 Route 108, Ste. D, Columbia, MD 21045; Great AAP; interested in programs importing data, reporting job availability, salary analysis, and management communication.

Biddle & Associates, Incorporated: 2100 Northrop Avenue, Suite 200, Sacramento, CA 95825-3937; EEO/AAP Analysis Software; Showing adverse impact analysis with import capacity for large databases such as 1996 census.

Criterion Incorporated: 9425 N. MacArthur Blvd, Irving, TX 75063; CAAMS; Generates reports for compliance plans and monitoring/managing multi-level reports.

Yocom and McKee, Incorporated: 15401 W. 9th Avenue, Golden, CO 80401; The Complete AAP, Employment Tracker; Produces analysis of census data, availability data, and tracking employment activity.

Attendance

Analytical Science Corporation: 10121 S. Ridgeland, Chicago Ridge, IL 60415; Electronic Payroll Management; calculates and tracks employee time, attendance, and work performance.

IMB: 18 Hurley Street, Cambridge, MA 02141; People Planner Schedule Manager, People-Planner Time & Attendance; Window-based programs for scheduling employee services, utilization, collection of employee attendance.

InTime Systems International: Centurion Tower Limited, 1601 Forum Place, Fifth floor, West Palm Beach, FL 33401; TAMS Time & Attendance Management System; Consolidates time, attendance entries from multiple collection sources, from payroll processing to database of historical company information.

Konetix Incorporated: 3210 Valmont Road, Boulder, CO 80301; TimeCentre; Custom and packaged solutions for remote and automated timekeeping and communication, with export capacities for interface with other computers.

Lathem Time Corporation: 200 Selig Drive, SW, Atlanta, GA 30336; Payclock for Windows; Software that allows user to track attendance and functions for employees.

Attitude Surveys

National Computer Systems Incorporated: 4401 W. 76th Street, Edina, MN 55435; NCS Survey; Window-based program design of surveys and scanning abilities for statistical reports.

Saja Software, Incorporated: 1490 Redwood Avenue, Boulder, CO 80304; Survey Select; User-friendly software to develop, administer, and analyze employee and customer responses

Scantron Corporation: 1361 Valencia Avenue, Tustin, CA 92680; PulseSurvey II, ScanSurvey; Report and survey generating with data analysis software allowing for processing, interpreting, and printing results in different categories.

Benefits Administration

ADP: 1 ADP Blvd., Roseland, NJ 07068; ADP/con; Software manufacturers of benefit planning, fringes, employee enrollment forms, and data.

Baker, Thomsen Associates: 901 Dove Street, Suite 158, Newport Beach, CA 92660; Benefit Assessor; Provides cost analyses, benefit statements, and produces application forms.

Benefit Plan Systems Corporation: 16 Technology Drive Suite 161, Irvine, CA 92718; COBRA EAS, Group Insurance Billing System; Software for processing and notification of benefits programs, with varying interface components for office networking.

Computer Communications Specialists Incorporated: 6529 Jimmy Carter Blvd., Nocross, GA 30071; First Line; Integrated software programs that converts touchtone telephone into a terminal for information transmission.

Coopers & Lybrand, LCP: 1301 Avenue of the Americas, New York, NY 10019; Retirement Counselor, Integrated Benefits Administration; Easy-to-use retirement planning software estimating income and expenses and software consolidating benefit options and savings.

DATAIR Employee Benefit Systems, Incorporated: 735 N. Cass Avenue, Westmont, IL 60559-1100; Flexible Benefit Systems; Enrollment tracking, division of cafeteria programs and complex mail mergers.

Dun & Bradstreet Software: 66 Perimeter Center E, Atlanta, CA 30346; TotalHR Personnel; Manages comprehensive employee data, retirement, and tracks health benefit utilization.

Flex Compensation Incorporated: 10405 6th Avenue, N. Suite 170 Plymouth, MN 55441; FlexAdmin-Election Enrollment Recordkeeping; Software designed produce personalized benefit enrollment forms, reimbursement accounts, and tracking of fringe utilization.

FLX Corporation: 301 Lindenwood Drive, Malvern, PA 19355; Visual HR Benefits Manager; Tracks employee coverages and calculates employee and employer costs with multiple-rate tables, and reporting capacities.

Genelco Incorporated: 1600 S. Brentwood Blvd, St. Louis, MO 63144-1330; Benefit Administration Plus; Supports billing, collections, and administration of group health plans with extensive, categorical reporting software.

GENESYS: 5 Branch Street, Methuen, MA 01844; Benefits Administration System; System separates and reports on different types of benefit plans (e.g., defined benefits, flexible benefits, etc.).

Compensation

Anchor Software Incorporated: 4966 El Camino Rael, Suite 216, Los Altos, CA 94022-1406; Total Comp; Compensation package analyzes job profiles, salary planning, market comparisons, and generating reports.

ERI Economic Research Institute: 16770 NE 79th Suite 104, Redmond, WA 98052; Salary Assessor, Geographic Assessor; Comparative statistical analysis on salary/wage distribution among different industries, U.S. and Canadian cities, and integrated with previous surveys.

Nardoni Associates Incorporated: 1465 Route 31, Annandale, NJ 08801; IncentiveComp; Windows-based system to set up incentive programs, with single and multiple performance measures, business results, and interfacing capacities with other databases.

Schroeder Associates: 3120 Masters Drive, Clearwater, FL 34621; SalesCom; Designed for sales force providing employee compensation data, policies, and specifications for commission earnings scale.

Computer-Based Training

Avator International Incorporated: Technology Park/Atlanta, 303 Research Drive, Suite 200, Nacross, GA 30092; Performance Systems Support Software; Microsoft-based program for customer service, leadership, total quality management training, with electronic support.

Compliance Software Incorporated: 6699 N. Landmark Drive, Suite A-157, Park City, UT 84098; Aware Drug & Alcohol Training; Interactive software designed for alcohol and drug prevention training with employee-awareness steps supplementing each unit.

Graphic Media Incorporated: 411 SW Second Avenue, Portland, OR 97204; ErgoKnowledge; One-hour interactive course teaching principles of healthy office ergonomics.

Innovus Corporation: 2060 E 2100 South, Salt Lake City, UT 84109; Innovus Multimedia; Multimedia development tool for creating easily modifiable business applications connected to corporate databases and able to be deployed over networks.

Park City Group: Main Street, Box 5000, Park City, UT 84060; InteractiveTutor; On-line training done at self-pace integrated with a central server, on varying training subjects.

Presenting Solutions Incorporated: 168 Santa Clara Avenue, Oakland, CA 94610; BrushUp; Computer-based training for over 30 software applications for Windows and Macintosh using simulated programs.

SHL KEE Systems: 10025 Governor Warfield Pkwy., Suite 400, Columbia, MD 21044; Computer Assisted Instructions; Computer-run curricula worked over network at employee's own pace.

Interviewing

Computer Employment Applications Incorporated: 606 W. Wisconsin Avenue, Suite 609, Milwaukee, WI 53203-1905; Preemployment interview system; Structured job interview protocol to get detailed, accurate information from application, with filing and storage systems.

Job Analysis and Assessment

Avantos: 5900 Hollis Street, Suite A, Emeryville,CA 94608; Avantos; Customized performance appraisal software for managers to write effective evaluations and improve appraisal process.

Development Dimensions International: 1225 Washington Pike, Bridgeville, PA 15017-2838; SynergEASE; User-friendly software analyzing critical competencies, job descriptions, multi-rater feedback, and generates evaluation performance measures.

Saville & Holdsworth Limited: 575 Boylston Street, Boston, MA 02116; Work Profiling System; Integrated job analysis and job evaluation software including task analysis, assessment methods, interview questions, person-job match, and point-factor matrix.

Success Factor Systems, Incorporated: One Embarcadero Center, Suite 2260, San Francisco, CA 94111; SFP 2000; Supports various competency models for assessment, development planning, performance management, and providing structured interview components.

Performance Management

Austin-Hayne Corporation: 2000 Alameda de las Pulgas, Suite 242, San Mateo, CA 94403; Employee Appraiser; Allows use of company's evaluation tools converted into database for monitoring performance and memo generation.

FEEDBACK PLUS: 5055 N.12th Street, Phoenix, AZ 85014; Interactive Feedback Network; Windows-based applicator for customized on-line employee assessments, producing individual and demographic reports.

Quality Coach Incorporated: PO Box 546, Nyack, NY 10960; PeopleBoard; Software for team performance management and appraisals, including project ratings and tracking.

Scott Hinshberger Associates: 3246 Wexford Circle, Idaho Falls 83404; PAF-360; Collects and reports degree performance feedback on people and organizations.

TEAMS Incorporated: 4450 S. Rural Road, Suite A-200, Tempe, AZ 85282; 360Feedback; Window-based client-server program allowing on-line support 24 hrs.

Resume and Job-Skills Tracking

Advanced Information Management Incorporated: 58 1/2 E. Burlington Avenue, Fairfield, IA 52556; HR Enterprise; Industrial-strength career tracking of employee service for different departments within an organization.

Best Program Incorporated: Abra Products Division, 888 Executive Center Drive W., St. Petersburg, FL 33702; Abra Recruiting; Software captures information from other Abra company software, organizes data, schedules reports, and updates efficiency of recruiting efforts.

Exxis Corporation: 207 Floral Vale, Yardley, PA 19067; Exxis Recruiting & Retension Management Systems; Database integrating applicant tracking, job-matches, employment requisitions, and different educational requirements, with best application in healthcare/hospitals.

Greentree Systems Incorporation: 201 San Antonio Circle #120, Mountain View, CA 94040; Greentree Employment Systems; Full-featured employment system with resume scanning and processing document imaging for applicant assessment.

Human Resource MicroSystems: 160 Sansome Street, Suite 1050; San Francisco, CA 94104; ATS-PRO; Tracks job requisition and applicants' qualifications, using report writer and library for references.

PowerMatch: 625 Ellis Street, Suite 303; Mountain View, CA 94043; PowerMatch; Stores faxed, scanned and e-mailed resumes, full text search and retrieval capabilities, interview, and requisition management with recruiting efforts prioritized.

Restrac Incorporated: 3 Allied Drive, Dedham, MA 02026; Restrac Hire; Advanced staffing system for application resources and selection, with basic features on resume data management and internet networking.

Resumix Incorporated: 890 Ross Drive, Sunnyvale, CA 94089; Resumix; Automates corporate staffing activities, using resume scanning and artificial intelligence technology.

Testing and Assessment

Bigby, Havis & Associates, Incorporated: 12750 Merit Drive, Suite 660, Dallas, TX; ASSESS; Expert system of full psychological assessment for selection, development, and career management including key points for interview probes and management recommendations.

Computerprep Incorporated: 410 N. 44th Street, Suite 600, Phoenix, AZ 85008-9880; PrepSkill Assessor; Computer skill assessment software designed to test, analyze, score, and define the strengths and weaknesses of employee software skills.

Know It All: 1530 Locust Street, Suite B/C, Philadelphia, PA 19102; Prove It Testing; Software assessing applicant and employee proficiency in over 40 popular software applications and office skills including on Word, WordPerfect, and Excel.

QWIZ Incorporated: 120 W. Wieuca Road, Suite 101, Atlanta, GA 30342; QWIZ; PC-based testing and training for typing, data entry, and applications of DOS, Windows platforms.

Training and Development

HTG: 280 Daine, Suite 200, Birmingham, MI 48809; TRIM; Manages training records, develops curricula, schedules training, and creates comprehensive reports for compliance to government standards (e.g., OSHA).

PSG International: One Blue Hill Plaza, Suite 1800, Pearl River, NY 10965; SPARQ Training; Windows software designed for database interface with course inventory and curriculum development options.

Silton-Bookman Systems: 20230 Stevens Creek Blvd., Suite D, Cupertino, CA 9501-5591; Registrar; Training administration system to register, track, and examine trainees with report writing on individual performance appraisals.

General Retail Software Companies

(**name:** address; contact;fax;phone;products;product description and needs)

Expert Software: 800 Douglas Road, North Tower, Suite 355, Coral Gables, FL 33134-3128; Khan Lowe; fax: 305-443-0786; phone: 305-567-9990; DOS games and Windows special-interest products appearing more in Radio Shack, Best Buy, and similar department stores.

Goodtimes Software: 1035 Dallas SE, Grand Rapids, MI 49507-1407; Dave Snyder, MVP Software; fax: 616-245-3204; phone: 616-245-8376; Mass distributed in Wal-Mart and other department stores in children's educational software.

Sofsource: 3186 Pine Tree Road, Lansing, MI 48911-4205; Rick Trask; phone: 517-393-8197; Personal Companion, Pro One; Focuses on exclusive contract on multihealth software.

UAV Corporation: PO Box 7647, Charlotte, NC 28241; Jeff Taylor; fax: 803-548-3335; phone: 803-548-7300; video and software products; Distribution in niche of inexpensive interactive games.

Villa Crespo Software: 501 South First Avenue, Suite L, Arcada, CA 91006; Donna L. Corson; phone: 708-433-0500; Coffee-Break; Specializes in under-$10 games for mass market.

TELEVISION PRODUCERS

Each of the entries below follows a sequence of information completed based on the replies from each producer or cable company or culled from a variety of different resources. Entirely completed entires include these items (unless shown differently under each heading):

Name of company: address, city, state, zip code; contact person; fax number; e-mail or URL (web page) address.

Industrial and Training Video Producers

Acclaim: 5200 Lankershim Blvd., North Hollywood, CA 91601-3100; Paul Carlin, Senior Staff Editor; fax: 818-752-5917.

Advantage Media Incorporated: 21356 Nordhoff Street, Suite 102, Chatsworth, CA 91311; Susan Cherno, Vice President; fax: 818-700-0612.

American Video Group Incorporated: 12020 W. Pico Blvd., Los Angeles, CA 90064-1127; fax: 310-473-5299.

Associated Audio/Video & Digital: 914 Arctic Street, Bridgeport, CT 06608; Richard Kraus, President.

A/V Concepts Corporation: 30 Montauk Blvd., Oakdale, NY 11769-1399; P. Solimene, President; fax: 516-567-8745.

Blate Associates: 10331 Watkins Mill Drive, Gaithersburg, MD 20879-2935; Samuel Blate, President; fax: 301-840-2248.

Cambridge Educational: 90 MacCorkle Avenue, SW, South Charleston,WV 205303; Charlotte Angel.

Center for Video Education: 56 Lafayette Avenue, North White Plains, NY 10603; President; fax: 914-428-0180.

Clearvue Incorporated: Dept. WM, 6465 N. Avondale Avenue, Chicago, IL 60631-1909; Mark Ventling, President; fax: 312-775-9844.

Continental Film Productions Corporation: PO Box 5126, 4220 Amnicola Hwy., Chattanooga, TN 37406; James Webster, President; fax: 615-629-0853.

Creative Productions: 1850 Redondo Avenue #104, Signal Hill, CA 90804-1251; Debora Castro; fax: 310-985-1365.

CRM Films: 2215 Faraday Avenue, Carlsbad, CA 92008; Peter Jordan, President; fax: 619-931-5792

DBM Publishing: a division of Drake, Beam Morin, Incorporated, 100 Park Avenue, New York, NY 10017; Director of Development; fax: 212-953-0194.

Development Dimensions International: 1225 Washington Pike, Bridgeville, PA 15017; President; fax: 412-257-0614.

Educational Insights: Editorial Dept., 19560 S. Rancho Way, Dominguez Hills, CA 90220; Livian Perez, Submissions Editor; fax: 310-605-5048.

Educational Video Network: 1401 19th Street, Huntsville, TX 77340; Dr. Kenneth Russell, President.

Edward Pacio & Associates: 26931 Deerweed Trail, Agoura Hills, CA 91301-5317; Edward Pacio, President; fax: 818-880-1586.

Effective Communication Arts Incorporated: PO Box 250, Wilton, CT 06897-0250; David Jacobson, President; fax: 203-761-0568.

The Film House Incorporated: 130 E. Sixth Street, Cincinnati, OH 45202; Ken Williamson, President.

Gears Communication: 120 S. Victory Blvd., Suite 202, Burbank, CA 91502-2801; Nadine Johnson; fax: 818-840-9358.

Gosch Productions: 1010 N. Lima Street, Burbank, CA 91505-2531; Pat Gosch; FAX: 818-843-7120.

Hayes School Publishing Company Incorporated: 321 Pennwood Avenue, Wilkinsburg, PA 15221-3398; Clair N. Hayes III, President; fax: 412-371-6408.

Informedia: PO Box 13287, Austin, TX 78711-3287; M. Sidoric, President.

Interactive Arts: 3200 Airport Avenue, Santa Monica, CA 90405; David Schwartz, Vice President.

Inter-Image Productions: 15910 Ventura Blvd., 10th Floor, Encino, CA 91436-2802; David Collins; fax: 818-995-6093.

Jerry Day Productions: 634 N. Reese Place, Burbank, CA 91506-1822; Jerry Day; fax: 818-843-3687.

Karr Production: 2925 W. Indian School Road, PO Box 11711, Phoenix, AZ 85017; President; fax: 602-266-4198.

Lewis Lipstone Productions: 5627 Sepulveda Blvd., Suite 204, Van Nuys, CA 91411-2920; Lewis Lipstone; fax: 818-994-5114.

Marina Beach Productions Incorporated: 520 Washington Blvd., #395, Marina Del Rey, CA 90292-5442; Scott Dobbie.

Media International: 5900 San Fernando Road, Glendale, CA 91202-2765; John Hasbrouck; fax: 818-242-5383.

Motivation Media Incorporated: 1245 Milwaukee Avenue, Glenview, IL 60025-2499; Kevin Kivikko, Senior Creative Director; fax: 708-297-6829.

Omni Productions: 655 W. Carmel Drive, Carmel, IN 46032-2500; Dr. Sandra Long, Vice-President.

Palardo Productions: 1807 Taft Avenue, Suite 4, Hollywood, CA 90028; Paul Ardolino, Director; fax: 213-469-8991.

Palo/Haklar & Associates: 650 N. Bronson Avenue, #144, Los Angeles, CA 90004-1404; Peter Haklar; fax: 213-465-2686.

Personnel Decisions International: 2000 Plaza VII Tower, 45 S. Seventh Street, Minneapolis, MN 55402; President; fax: 612-337-8292.

Photo Communication Services, Incorporated: 6055 Robert Drive, Traverse City, MI 49684; M. Lynn Hartwell, President.

Schleger Company: 200 Central Park S., 27-B, New York, NY 10019-1415; Peter Schleger, President; fax: 212-245-4973.

Slingshot Productions: 8309 Ponce Avenue, Canoga Park, CA 91304-3336; Allesandro Machi; fax: 818-999-2539.

SMS Film & Video Productions: 8544 Sunset Blvd., West Hollywood, CA 90069-210; Lisa Shanks; fax: 310-652-3322.

Stuart Rowlands & Associates, Incorporated: 3132 La Surviva Drive, Los Angeles, CA 90068; Stuart Rowlands; fax: 213-850-6138.

Talco Productions: 279 E. 44th Street, New York, NY 10017-4354; Alan Lawrence, President; fax: 212-697-4827.

Tar Associates Incorporated: 230 Venie Way, Venice, CA 90291; Ed Tar, President; fax: 310-306-0654.

Tel-Air Associates, Incorporated: 1755 NE 149th Street, Miami, FL 33181; Grant Gravitt, President; fax: 305-944-1143.

Ultitech, Incorporated: Foot of Broad Street, Stratford, CT 06497; President; fax: 203-375-6699; e-mail: comcowic@world. std.com.

United Training Media: 6633 W. Howard Street, PO Box 48718, Nile, IL 60714-0718; President; fax: 708-647-0918.

Verne Pershing Productions: 524 E. Marigold Street, Alta Dena, CA 91009-1545; Verne Pershing; fax: 213-464-2610.

Video Arts Incorporated: 8614 W. Catalpa Avenue, Chicago, IL 60656; Producer; fax: 312-693-7030.

Video Resources: PO Box 18642, Irvine, CA 92713; Brad Hagen, President.

Visual Horizons: 180 Metro Park, Rochester, NY 14623; Stanley Feingold, President; fax: 716-424-5313.

Widget Productions Limited: 120 Duane Street, #8, New York, NY 10007; Tery Krueger.

Infomerical and Commerical Video Producers

American Marketing Systems: 6951 High Grove Blvd., Burr Ridge, IL 60521; Clifford Rose, Director of Marketing; fax: 708-325-0825.

Amherst Entertainment Incorporated: 8 Glen Drive, South Salem, NY 10590-2309; Brian Benlifer, President; fax: 914-533-6193.

Apsicon Productions, Incorporated: 9600 Kirkside Road Los Angeles, CA 90035-4010; Angela Schapiro, Producer; fax: 310-558-0121.

Ben Kalb Productions: 1341 Ocean Avenue, #160, Santa Monica, CA 90401-1066; Ben Kalb; fax: 310-820-9768.

Big Picture Shows: 15 W. 44th Street, New York, NY 10036; Ava Seavey, Director of Marketing; fax: 212-768-3907.

Bosustow Media Group: 7655 Sunset Blvd., Suite 114, Hollywood, CA 90046-2700; Tee Bosustow, Producer; fax: 213-851-5599.

Catalina Entetainment Group Incorporated: 5751 Buckingham Pkwy., Culver City, CA 90230-6521; John Fondy; fax: 310-216-0056.

Concepts Video Productions: 170 Changebridge Road, Montville, NJ 07045; Collette Liantonio, President; fax: 201-808-5623.

Cummings Entertainment Group: 20329 Arminta Street, Canoga Park, CA 91306; Drew Cummings, President; fax: 818-701-9494.

Direct Hit Productions: 3 Piedmont Center, Suite 300, Atlanta, GA 30305; Ellen Cross, President; fax: 404-233-0302.

Film Factory: 9845 Santa Monica Blvd., Beverly Hills, CA 90212; Bob Alexander, Producer; fax: 310-551-3041; e-mail: telegence@earthlink.net.

Five Star Productions: 5301 N. Federal Hwy., Boca Raton, FL 33487; Scott Woolley, Executive Producer; fax: 407-997-9660; e-mail: fivestar@emi.net; website: http://www.vstar.com/.

Four Point Entertainment: 3575 Cahuenga Blvd., West, Suite 600, Los Angeles, CA 90068; Julie Resh, Vice-President Development of Productions; fax: 213-850-6709.

Frederiksen Television Incorporated: 2735 Hartland Road, Suite 300, Falls Church, VA 22043; Lee Fredericksen, President; fax: 703-560-8292.

Galanty & Company: 1640 5th Street, Suite 202; Santa Monica, CA 90401-3388; Mark Galanty, Executive Producer; fax: 310-451-5020.

Gerren Productions: 3640 W. 63rd Street, Suite 1A, Los Angeles, CA 90043; Conrad Bullard, Vice President of Productions; fax: 213-293-8214.

Goldberg & O'Reily: 1551 S. Robertson Blvd., Suite 102, Los Angeles, CA 90035-4257; Spike Jones; fax: 310-556-1658.

Gunfor Hire Film & Tape: 3019 Pico Blvd., Santa Monica, CA 90405-2003; Alan Stamm, Editor; fax: 310-315-1757.

Guthy-Renker Television (and Productions): 3340 Ocean Park Blvd., 2nd floor, Santa Monica, CA 90405; Michael Wex, President; fax: 310-581-3232.

Hanheld Productions: 421 N. Rodeo Drive #15295, Beverly Hills, CA 90210-4500; Mona McCartney, Producer; fax: 310-777-0402.

Hawthorne Communications: 300 N. 16th Street, Fairfield, IA 52556; Time Hawthorne, President; fax: 515-472-6043.

Hokus Pokus Productions Incorporated: 2290 Ventura Blvd., Suite 265, Woodland Hills, CA 91364-1204; Robert Haukoos; fax: 818-224-2054.

Horton Associates, Incorporated: 2020 Alameda Padre Serra, Suite 223; Santa Barbara, CA 93103; Andrew Horton, Vice President, Production; fax: 805-963-3157; e-mail: tha@sharktv.com; webpage: http://www.sharktv.com.

Howard Productions, Incorporated: 1040 N. Las Palmas, #236, Los Angeles, CA 90038; Al Howard, President, Executive Producer; fax: 213-960-2531.

ICN Productions: 12401 W. Olympic Blvd., Los Angeles, CA 90064-1022; Ruth Flores; fax: 310-447-7906.

If/X Productions: 3522 Knobhill Drive, Sherman Oaks, CA 91423; Bruce Tiplett, Vice President, Development; fax: 818-501-4526.

In-Finn-Ity Productions, Incorporated: 345 N. Maple Drive, #184, Beverly Hills, CA 90210-3827; Terry Finn; fax: 310-777-0110.

Info Marketing Group: 1936 La Mesa Drive, Santa Monica, CA 90402-2323; Bill Flohr, President; fax: 310-394-6934.

Infomercial Solutions: 5512 Meadow Vista Way, Agoura Hills, CA 91301-1507; Rosemary Kavanaugh; fax: 818-879-1148.

In Sync Productions Incorporated: PO Box 64755, Virginia Beach, VA 23467; Nancy Kondas, President; fax: 804-460-1927.

Kent & Spiegel Direct Incorporated: 6133 Bristol Pkwy., Suite 150, Culver City, CA 90230-6613; fax: 310-337-1011.

Kobs & Draft Worldwide: 142 E. Ontario, Chicago, IL 60611; Howard Draft, Chairman; fax: 312-944-3566.

Lance Douglas Direct Response: 402 Calle Miramar, Redondo Beach, CA 90277-6442; Lance Douglas; fax: 310-373-9645.

McNamara & Associates: 5301 Calhoun Avenue, Sherman Oaks, CA 91401-5712; Jim McNamara, President; fax: 818-907-8032.

Moffitt Associates: 747 N. Lake Avenue, Pasadena, CA 91104; Lynne Moffitt, Executive Producer; fax: 818-791-3092; e-mail: jvtm55a@prodigy.com.

Onyx Productions Incorporated: 8218 Melrose Avenue, Suite 201, Los Angeles, CA 90046-6812; Joan Mellini-Renfrow; fax: 213-653-8975.

Paige Associates, Incorporated: 3000 W. Olympic Blvd., Suite 1407, Santa Monica, CA 90404-5041; George Paige, President; fax: 310-315-4836.

Pantron One Corporation: 8322 Beverly Blvd., Los Angeles, CA 90048-2600; Jason Graves; fax: 213-655-7199.

Paradigm Communication Group: 250 Production Plaza, Cincinnati, OH 45219; Bill Speigel, President; fax: 513-381-8756.

Paraview Incorporated: 1674 Broadway, Suite 4B, New York, NY 10019; Sandra Martin, Executive Producer; fax: 212-489-5371.

Positive Response Television: 14724 Ventura Blvd., Suite 600, Sherman Oaks, CA 91403-3501; Gary Hewitt; fax: 818-380-6966.

Power Media Markeitng Group: 150 East Olive Avenue, Suite 305, Burbank, CA 91502; Gene Williams or Leeann Johnson; fax: 818-557-8318.

The Production Partners: 786 King Street W, Toronto, Ontario, Canada M5V 1N6; Ed Crain; fax: 416-363-4342.

Total Eclipse Productions: 11714 Canton Place, Studio City, CA 91604; Randy Callaham, Executive Producer; fax: 818-754-0971; e-mail: callahan@aol.com.

Transactional Media Incorporated: 345 N. Maple Drive #205, Beverly Hills, CA 90210-3827; Earl Greenberg; fax: 310-571-3510.

Tri-Crown Productions: 3900 W. Alameda Avenue, Suite 700, Burbank, CA 91505; Dan Weyand, Vice-President, Production and Program Development; fax: 818-955-7338.

Two-D Productions: 953 N. Highland Avenue, Los Angeles, CA 90068; Michael McGahee, President; fax: 213-850-5015.

Tyee Productions: 513 NW 13th Avenue, 5th Floor, Portland, OR 97209; John Ripper, President; fax: 503-228-0560.

Videoworks: 3435 Ocean Park Blvd., Suite 208, Santa Monica, CA 90405-3314; David Werk; fax: 310-839-5603.

Washington Media Works: 708 North Wayne Street, Suite 205, Arlington, VA 22201; Kenneth White, Executive Vice President; fax: 703-525-0658.

Western Direct Response: 8544 Sunset Blvd., Los Angeles, CA 90069; Darrel Griffin, Executive Vice President; fax: 310-854-7558.

Williams Television Time: 3130 Wilshire Blvd., 4th Floor, Santa Monica, CA 90403-2304; Kathleen Williams, President; fax: 310-829-4454.

Zemi The Film and Video Company: 2718 Lake Hollywood Drive, Los Angeles, CA 90068; Victoria Powells-Conway, President; fax: 213-957-9220; e-mail: vicon@aol.com.

New TV Cable Networks

(**Network:** address; key personnel; fax; phone; description.)

ACCESS TELEVISION NETWORK: 2062 Business Center Drive, Suite 230, Irvine, CA 92715; William Cullen, Chairman; fax: 714-757-1526; phone: 714-442-6170; Infomercial programming service.

THE AIR & SPACE NETWORK: 2701 NW Vaughn Street, Suite 475, Portland, OR 97210-5366; Matthew Simek, CEO; fax: 503-241-3507; phone: 503-224-9821; Pay service on aviation and space-themed programming.

AMERICA'S COLLECTIBLES NETWORK: 1614 Industrial Road, PO Box 2136; Greeneville, TN 37744-2135; Bill Kourns, Vice President, Programming;

fax: 423-639-5082; phone: 423-639-5611; Home shopping service featuring gems, coins, and jewelry.

AMERICA'S HEALTH NETWORK: 1000 Universal Studios Plaza, Bldg. 22A, Orlando, FL 32819-7617; George Hulcher, Vice President, Programming; phone: 407-345-8555; Health information channel, using call-in format.

AMERICA'S TALKING: 2200 Fletcher Avenue, Ft. Lee, NJ 07024; Beth Tilson, Vice President, Programming; fax: 201-346-2141; phone: 346-6777; Live, interactive talk programming covering news and entertainment subjects.

ANIMAL PLANET: 7700 Wisconsin Avenue, Bethesda, MD 20814-3579; fax: 301-986-4628; phone: 301-986-0444; Documentary channel featuring animal and natural history topics.

ANIMAL/VISION: THE ANIMAL CHANNEL: 24 Fifth Avenue, Suite 1219, New York, NY 10011; Michael Du Monceau, Programming Co-principal; fax: 212-260-9204; phone: 212-529-0391; Fictional/nonfiction programming service with animal themes.

THE ANTI-AGING NETWORK: PO Box 3485, Beverly Hills, CA 90212; Lloyd Frerer, Co-partner, Programming Director; fax: 213-879-5923; phone: 310-277-4150; Network presenting cutting-edge health and anti-aging scientific advances.

THE ARTS & CRAFTS NETWORK: 200 Orchard Ridge Drive, Suite 215, Gaithersburg, MD 20878; George Verdier, Chairman; fax: 301-253-9620; phone: 800-210-9900; Arts and crafts oriented network, including how-to, studio tours, interviews, and home shopping segments.

ARTS & ANTIQUES NETWORK: National Press Building, Suite 2003, Washington, DC 20045; Douglas Ritter, President; fax: 202-347-1342; phone: 703-553-0472; Niche service devoted to arts, antiques, cultural heritage, and preservation and restoration auction activity.

THE AUTO CHANNEL: 624 W. Main Street, 6th Floor, Louisville, KY 40202; Mark Rauch, Executive Vice President; fax: 502-568-2501; phone: 800-584-4105; News and entertainment service featuring coverage of automotive products and motorsports.

AUTOMOTIVE TELEVISION NETWORK: 274 Great Road, Acton, MA 01720; John Coscia, Senior Vice President, Programming; fax: 508-264-9547; phone: 508-264-9921; Car and motorsports programming.

THE BENEFIT NETWORK: 8033 Sunset Blvd., Suite 579, West Hollywood, CA 90046; Barbara Peck, President; fax: 310-559-7550; phone: 310-452-5339; Education and entertainment service that benefits global humanitarian and ecology causes.

THE BOATING CHANNEL: 135 W. 87th Street, Studio A, New York, NY 10024-2903; Madeline Amgott, Executive Vice President, Programming; fax:

212-787-5253; phone: 212-877-0500; Marine news, information, and entertainment.

BOOKNET: 45 Rockefeller Plaza, 20th Floor, New York, NY 10111; Burton Pines, President; fax: 212-698-2472; phone: 212-698-7808; A showcase of the latest books in every genre, with on-air tie-ins.

CAREER & EDUCATION OPPORTUNITY NETWORK: 201 Santa Monica Blvd., Suite 400, Santa Monica, CA 90401; R. Anthony Cort, Chairman; fax: 310-393-1147; phone: 310-451-0451; Information and motivational service, presenting career and educational opportunities.

THE CEO CHANNEL: 8 Allerman Road, Oakland, NJ 07436; Neil Sheridsam, Executive Vice President; fax: 516-626-7548; phone: 516-626-7730; Magazine-style service presenting programs of interest to the world's corporate leaders.

CHILDREN'S CABLE NETWORK: 801 S. Main Street, Burbank, CA 91506; Patricia Moore, Vice President, Production; fax: 818-556-6363; phone: 818-556-6300; Entertainment and educational service for pre-school children.

CHOP TV: 3283 Motor Avenue, 2nd floor, Los Angeles, CA 90034; Steve Beebe, Executive in charge of programming; fax: 310-841-6965; phone: 310-841-6964; Martial arts network presented in a magazine style format.

COMPUTER NETWORK: 150 Chestnut Street, San Francisco, CA 94111; Dan Sexton, Vice President, Development; fax: 415-395-9205; phone: 415-395-7800; Programming about computers, on-line, and interactive media developments.

COLLECTORS CHANNEL: 67 River Street, PO Box 702, Hudson, MA 01749; Fred Sherman, Vice President, Programming; fax: 508-562-1196; phone: 508-568-0856; Programming service targeted to collectors of various merchandise and memorabilia.

CONSERVATIVE TELEVISION NETWORK: 801 N. Fairfax Street, Suite 312, Alexandria, VA 22314; Jeb Spencer, Vice President, Network Development; fax: 703-739-0664; phone: 703-836-3257; News,information and entertainment from conservative perspectives.

CONSUMER RESOURCE NETWORK: PO Box 989, Equinox Junior Bldg., 2nd Floor, Manchester, VT 05254; John Engel, Business Development Director; fax: 802-362-5401; phone: 802-362-0505; Information channel covering new consumer products and services.

THE DREAM NETWORK: 8115 Fenton Street, Suite 100, Silver Spring, MD 20910; Alvin Jones, President; fax: 301-588-0208; phone: 301-565-5948; Urban audience-oriented service, emphasizing news, talk, music video, and inspirational programs.

THE ECOLOGY CHANNEL: 1660 Soldiers Field Road, Boston, MA 02135; Netty Douglas, Ecxecutive Vice President, Programming-Operations; fax: 410-465-9672; phone: 410-750-7291; Service covering people, ideas, and issues related to the environment.

THE ENRICHMENT CHANNEL: 145 Avenue of the Americas, 2nd Floor, New York, NY 10013; Michael Schwager, President; fax: 212-627-8733; phone: 212-366-1841; Programming on human potential, self-help, and community outreach services.

THE EPIC CHANNEL: 1020 15th Street, Suite 19J, Denver, CO 80202; David Hill, President, fax: 303-892-9419; phone: 303-892-9418; Programming network offering information and entertainment series on money, sex, and power.

FASHION & DESIGN TELEVISION: 375 N. Greenwich Street, New York, NY 10013; Anthony Guccione II, President; fax: 212-941-3874; phone: 212-941-3990; American and international fashion, design, travel, and entertainment trends.

FASHION NETWORK: 226 W. 26th Street, New York, NY 10001; James Deutch, President; fax: 212-462-4551; phone: 212-462-4500; Fashion news and information service.

FIT CABLE: 2877 Guardian Lane, Virginia Beach, VA 23452; Jake Steinfeld, Programming Director; fax: 804-459-6426; phone: 804-459-6000; Health and fitness, exercise, and lifestyle service.

FITNESS INTERACTIVE: 9220 Sunset Blvd., Suite 224, Los Angeles, CA 90069; Alan Mruvka, Co-chairman; fax: 310-271-3479; phone: 310-271-5400; Fitness and exercise network hosted by celebrities and top instructors.

GOLDEN AMERICAN NETWORK: 9250 Wilshire Blvd., Suite 412, Beverly Hills, CA 90212; Jim Gates, Vice President, Production; fax: 310-858-0321; phone: 310-858-1115; Service for people age 50 and over.

THE GOLF CHANNEL: 7580 Commerce Center Drive, Orlando, FL 32819; Robert Greenway, Senior Vice President, Programming-Operations; fax: 407-363-7976; phone: 407-363-4653; Golf-oriented channel, featuring event coverage from around the world.

THE GOSPEL NETWORK: 6430 Sunset Blvd, Suite 1400, Hollywood, CA 90028; Reginald Utley, Program Director; fax: 213-469-7516; phone: 213-469-4322; Gospel music, entertainment, and news service.

THE HISTORY CHANNEL: 235 E. 45th Street, New York, NY 10017; Abbe Raven, Senior Vice President, Programming-Production; fax: 212-210-9755; phone: 212-661-4500; Historical documentaries, movie, and miniseries program service.

HOBBY CRAFT NETWORK: 990 Highland Drive, Solana Beach, CA 92075; Rita Weiss, President; fax: 619-259-9632; phone: 619-259-2305; Hobby and craft programming using demonstrations and experts.

HOME & GARDEN TELEVISION NETWORK: 9701 Madison Avenue, Knoxville, TN 37932; Ed Spray, Senior Vice President, Programming-Production; fax: 423-531-8933; phone: 423-694-2700; How-to advice on home remodeling, repairs, decorating, and gardening.

JONES COMPUTER NETWORK: 9697 E. Mineral Avenue, Englewood, CO 80112; Robert Jones, Vice President, Programming; fax: 303-784-5608; phone: 303-792-3111; Programming that appeals to the spectrum of computer users.

JONES HEALTH NETWORK: 9697 E. Mineral Avenue, Englewood, CO 80112; Robert Jones, Vice President, Programming; fax: 303-792-5608; phone: 303-792-3111; Health education and information programming.

KID CITY: One Lincoln Plaza, New York, NY 10023; Douglas Lee, Senior Vice President; fax: 212-875-6114; phone: 212-595-3465; Educational service for kids ages 2 to 12.

THE LOVE NETWORK: 241 E. 58th Street, Suite 4D, New York, NY 10022; Josefina Gamundi, President; fax/phone: 212-752-4657; Personal relationship-oriented channel, focusing on self-esteem and improvement.

THE MILITARY CHANNEL: 101 Bullitt Lane, Suite 307, Louisville, KY 40222; Nancy Hoke, Programming Director; fax: 502-425-8597; phone: 502-429-0200; Network for military and aviation enthusiasts.

NATIVE AMERICAN NATIONS NETWORK: 107 Freeport Road, Pittsburgh, PA 15215; Eric Hughes, Vice President, Programming; fax: 412-782-4242; phone: 412-782-2921; Information and entertainment service geared to Native Americans.

NET–POLITICAL NEWSTALK NETWORK: 717 2nd Street, NE, Washington, DC 20002; Meryln Reineke, Program Director; fax: 202-546-0182; phone: 202-546-3200; Public policy and educational programming.

NEW SCIENCE NETWORK: PO Box 621165, Littleton, CO 80162; Phil Catalano, President; fax/phone: 303-575-6289; Programming devoted to new science breakthroughs.

THE OUTDOOR CHANNEL: 43445 Business Park Drive, Suite 103, Temecula, CA 92590; Claudia Wolfkind, Program Development Director; fax: 909-699-6313; 909-699-6991; Outdoor and recreational activity-oriented network.

PARENT TELEVISION: 966 Hilgard Avenue, Los Angeles, CA 90024; Debbie Myers, Senior Vice President, Programming; fax: 310-824-1150; phone: 310-824-0689; Service covering all aspects of parenting.

PARENTHOOD TELEVISION: 193 Lakewood Drive, Rockville Center, NY 11570; John Wheeler, President and CEO; fax: 516-763-4643; phone: 516-678-6017; Service focusing on child and parent development topics.

PARENTING SATELLITE TELEVISION NETWORK: 90 MacCorkle Avenue, SW., S. Charleston, WV 25303; Edward Gardner, CEO; fax: 800-329-6787; phone: 304-746-7786; Programs and home shopping segments for parents of children up to age 17.

THE PET TELEVISION NETWORK: 9230 Robin Drive, Los Angeles, CA 90069; Chris Wood, Executive Vice President, Production; fax: 310-550-0830;

phone: 310-550-7280; Entertainment and information service on pets, zoos, and wildlife.

PLANET CENTRAL TELEVISION: 6611 Santa Monica Blvd., Los Angeles, CA 90038; Tom Tatum, President; fax: 213-469-2193; phone: 213-871-2900; Altenative television channel covering ecology trends and issues.

PREMIERE HORSE NETWORK: 2740 W. Magnolia Blvd., Burbank, CA 91505; Chris Shelton, Senior Vice President, Programming; fax: 818-955-9051; phone: 818-955-9000; Premium channel covering equestrian, rodeo, and related events.

PRIME LIFE NETWORK: 2 Penn Plaza, New York, NY 10121; Linda Wendell, Vice President, Programming; fax: 212-868-8697; phone: 212-594-5050; Entertainment service catering to adults 50 years and up.

THE RECOVERY NETWORK: 206 N. Signal Street, Suite N, Ojai, CA 93023; Cis Wilson, Vice President, Programming; fax: 805-640-1665; phone: 805-640-1660; Service for people dealing with drug addiction, eating, and compulsive gambling disorders.

THE SINGLES NETWORK: 150 Crosways Park West, Woodbury, NY 11797; Laurie Gidins, Senior Vice President, Business Development; fax: 516-364-5948; phone: 516-364-5948; Lifestyle service for singles.

THE SPACE NETWORK: PO Box 2778, Rancho Mirage, CA 92270; Jules Ross, President; phone: 619-770-3474; Educational service covering astronomy, space exploration, and the humanities.

Index

Page numbers followed by the letter "i" indicate illustrations; those followed by the letter "t" indicate tables.